the first steps
to
FITNESS

How to Stop *Thinking* about It and Start *Doing* It

elizabeth williams

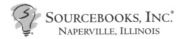
SOURCEBOOKS, INC.
NAPERVILLE, ILLINOIS

Published by Sourcebooks, Inc.
P.O. Box 4410, Naperville, Illinois 60567-4410
(630) 961-3900
FAX: (630) 961-2168
www.sourcebooks.com

Library of Congress Cataloging-in-Publication Data

Williams, Elizabeth M.
 First steps to fitness / by Elizabeth M. Williams.
    p. cm.
 ISBN 1-4022-0033-1 (alk. paper)
 1. Physical fitness. 2. Exercise. I. Title.
RA781.W495 2004
613.7—dc21

                              2004006158

                 Printed and bound in Canada
          WC 10 9 8 7 6 5 4 3 2 1

Dedication

I would like to dedicate *The First Steps to Fitness* to all of my personal training clients. Because of their openness and honesty, I saw the patterns and struggles that we shared. Because of their willingness to change and to accept challenges, I witnessed transformations. Because of their great spirit and courage, I was inspired to write this book.

Contents

Preface

For a long time, I seemed like the last person who would write a fitness book, especially one that contained a psychological and spiritual approach. For years, I wrestled with negative body image and an eating disorder, beat myself up with food and exercise, tried to get that perfect body, and was never satisfied. Only when I faced the insecurities and fears driving my negative behavior was I able to move beyond them. Later, having received a bachelor's degree in psychology and worked for several years as an aerobics instructor and personal trainer, I realized the importance of emotional factors on fitness success, not just in my life but in others'.

As a personal trainer, I found many clients had feelings and issues similar to mine. Some had been rejected or had feared rejection for not being thin, fit, or toned enough. Many admitted to over- or undereating for emotional reasons. Others were depressed about the way they looked, which made it difficult to gather the strength and will to work out, especially on a long-term basis.

Most were dissatisfied with their bodies, images, diets, and dress sizes, and could benefit by addressing the internal issues blocking them from external results.

Those clients who successfully established a fitness lifestyle shared certain characteristics. They had cultivated inner strength, self-motivation, maturity, self-discipline, faith, self-love, patience, and self-respect. In contrast, individuals who had not developed these qualities stopped exercising shortly after our sessions ended even though they had lost weight and inches, had become stronger, and felt better. Outward success wasn't enough. Inner change was necessary.

Some may believe they have no internal barriers to resolve. "I'm thirty pounds overweight because I ate too much, exercised too little, had a baby, started birth control, quit smoking, was injured on the job," or any number of reasons. We know we have to exercise and eat right and perhaps we do for a week or a month or even a year, but then we return to our old ways. Consistently, 60 to 70 percent of new exercisers quit within the first six months. Why?

Based on personal and professional experience working with hundreds of clients, I believe the fitness industry has approached fitness from a physiological standpoint while often ignoring psychological and spiritual factors. What are we thinking and feeling when we reach for that cheesecake or skip aerobics class for the second week in a row? What propels some to work out compulsively three hours a day and eat only a tiny salad for dinner?

For years, exercise psychologists have studied and have recognized the impact of psychological factors in staying fit, but many fitness centers have not embraced this research or used it to empower members. If they did, fewer members would leave soon after joining. Health clubs profit by signing people up on annual contracts billable whether members come to the gym or not.

With regular one-on-one contact with clients, personal trainers get to know their clients extremely well. Of the hundreds of personal trainers I've interviewed, the majority agree that in order for clients to succeed, their internal issues must be addressed. Some of these obstacles include low self-esteem, fear, insecurity, past fitness failures, boredom with exercise, depression, impatience, and negativity.

Another component to success is understanding your motives for becoming fit. Do you want to make yourself more attractive? Feel better in your clothes? Prove to an ex-boyfriend that he shouldn't have dumped you? Gain love and acceptance? Or are you simply tired of being tired? Tired of feeling fat? Tired of your waistband digging into your belly?

Initially, you may not be completely aware of what is compelling you to change. A common motive is to get fit to please someone else. This sets you up for disappointment and failure if that someone doesn't appreciate your effort. What if you do all this work to get fit so that your significant other will find you more attractive and three months later, after you've lost thirty pounds and gone down four sizes, he says, without looking up from the television, "Yeah, you look better. Now be quiet and pass me the popcorn." What happens to your motivation then? You might decide he's not worth it and go back to your old ways and gain the weight back, almost as a way to get back at him.

Some of your motives might be based on fear—fear of not getting what you want or losing what you have (love, pride, acceptance, success). The parent who tells her child that she is fat and should quit eating so much may be motivated by fear that others may not accept her child. The teenager who quits tap class may be acting out of fear of failure and inadequacy.

A wise friend, Anna, taught me, "Either you're coming from a place of love or you're coming from a place of fear." When most people would have curled into a ball and shouted, "I quit," Anna not only didn't give up when she found out she had HIV, she thrived. She became active in the community and with AIDS organizations and further developed a strong faith. Her internal strength comes from faith and love. She credits these beliefs for keeping her free of AIDS symptoms for the last fourteen years without having to take any HIV/AIDS drugs. She taught me that there are only two true emotions—love and fear. All the other emotions originate from one of these two. Are your motives based on love or fear?

So what if you have been motivated by fear? If it gets you to work out and eat healthfully, what else matters? People driven by fear eventually run out of gas and are usually miserable along the way. Dance because you love to dance, not because you think you're fat and want to lose weight before the reunion. Forgo the chocolate cake and have your favorite fruit instead, not because of fear of gaining weight but out love for your body. Work out because you want to be around to see your kids grow up, spend time with your spouse in old age, enjoy golf in your eighties.

As you work through this book, be honest with yourself, cultivate unconditional love, build inner strength, and challenge yourself—and you will have long-lasting fitness.

Tools:

Notebooks & Athletic Shoes

Begin by moving your body for twenty minutes or more every day. It doesn't matter whether it is a simple walk around the block or something more technical like martial arts. This activity isn't meant to torture you. You can have fun. You could go bike riding, dancing, or in-line skating. You can do the same thing every day or try something different each time. It doesn't matter, as long as you're moving. You're not attempting to burn one thousand calories in twenty minutes. You're practicing consistency. If you miss a day or two, just start back up as soon as possible. For this, and other activities that come later in the book, consider investing in a good pair of athletic shoes.

Read one or two chapters per week instead of rushing through them. Allow time to do some of the suggested writing exercises. It is time well spent. Writing helps people overcome stressful emotional experiences, maintain a positive attitude, and better understand themselves. The writing is for your eyes only, unless you choose to share it. Grammar, spelling, and even content are not important. Use a blank notebook, journal, or loose-leaf paper. Writing on the computer will suffice, but it tends to produce more rational, black-and-white material. Writing by hand more effectively engages emotions. The process brings together our whole selves: body (hand, fingers, shoulders), mind (thoughts), and soul (feelings). One study done at North Dakota State University showed a connection between writing and physical health. Medical patients who wrote about emotionally intense events had greater health improvements over four months than those who didn't.

Do as many of the assignments as you can. If pressed for time, choose the two or three that catch your attention first. Because fitness is a process, you may want to go through this book more than once and complete any assignments you skipped the first time.

Some readers may find that the assignments stir up more emotion than they can handle alone and may want to consider talking to a counselor or other professional.

To work this program most effectively, make a commitment—a decision followed by action. I don't enjoy making commitments any more than anyone else. But I've learned that to achieve anything worthwhile, it is necessary to commit to certain actions and remain consistent. Mary Kay Ash, the founder of Mary Kay Cosmetics, said, "Consistency is the key to success," and she knew, having created one of the most successful skin-care companies in the world.

The first step is making a decision, committing to yourself the time, energy, work, and patience to be your best. The next step is following that decision with action.

One client, Claire, made a commitment and achieved the seemingly impossible. In her mid-forties, she worked out every day and ate healthfully. She was happy with her slender body. Then Claire was sick for a week with the flu. Upon recovery, she began to have pain in her back that made exercise difficult. When the pain worsened, she went to see a doctor. After a few misdiagnoses and a year of unrelenting pain, she learned that the flu virus had settled in her spine. Her body was trying to kill the virus but in the process was destroying the nerves in her spine. By the time the doctors realized what was happening, she was almost completely paralyzed from the waist down. The doctors said she might never walk again, at least not without a cane or walker.

But Claire didn't accept defeat. She wanted to return to her active lifestyle. She couldn't imagine life without the activities she once enjoyed. She also wanted to lose the thirty pounds she had gained that year. Claire committed herself to doing whatever she had to do, including daily physical therapy. A year later, she was able to participate regularly in water aerobics.

I met Claire two years after she was told she would never walk again. Six feet tall and graceful, without a cane or walker, Claire strode into the gym lobby where I was waiting. She attributed her full recovery to determination, spiritual strength, and hard work. But she hadn't reached all of her goals yet. She wanted to gain strength and lose more weight through weight lifting and other exercises.

Several times pain forced her to take a week or two off. Others might have given up, but Claire didn't—because of her commitment. Whenever she suffered, she didn't feel sorry for herself. She planned her next step and sought solutions.

Although Claire's progress was slow, she prevailed. In contrast, other clients with no physical limitations struggled with negativity, frustration, and lack of motivation often because they weren't progressing as fast as they wanted. Unlike Claire, they were suffering from internal barriers, not external ones. As if they were victims, they were approaching fitness as something they *had* to do, rather than something they *chose* to do. I had less faith that these clients would reach and maintain fitness goals than Claire would, although they had every advantage.

Janet, another client, also made a commitment to working out and eating right no matter what happened in her daily life. With fifty pounds to lose, she suffered recurring colitis attacks that left her weak and tired. However, she committed herself to working out five or six days per week, and she did, even when she didn't feel like it. She often traveled for work but didn't allow her trips to stop her, exercising in her hotel room, bringing her own food to avoid eating fast food, and working out in whatever gym she could find. She steadily lost weight and inches and reached her goals.

How do you know if you've made a commitment? You forge ahead despite the distractions of the world. You go to the gym even when you feel like sitting on the couch. You follow a balanced eating plan even when you feel like eating a whole pie in one sitting. You follow your routine to the best of your ability no matter which way the wind is blowing.

You must have already made a preliminary decision to work toward greater fitness since you have read this far. Now, solidify your commitment to this exciting, life-changing process by making a written contract with yourself. Below is a contract to sign as a reminder of the commitment you've made (or write your own). Post your commitment where you can read it daily.

The First Steps to Fitness Commitment Contract

I, _____, have made the decision that I am ready to become more fit, and I am committed to doing the necessary actions. Also, as I work toward greater fitness, I will remain patient with myself and my progress.

Signed_____ Date_____

Now, armed with tools such as notebooks and athletic shoes, let's begin.

JOURNAL

Tell here your triumphs and delights.
Describe the sights and score the fights
which mark this day from any other.
Tell about your dad and mother.

Speak of your maybes and your mights,
and the joy of inspiration's heights.
Set all down here without a quiver
of censorship—your private river
to wash away regret and loss
and sift resentments' gritty dross.

Write about your moments tender
and tell about your fender bender.
Tell how it is—and how it seems.
Record your day and nighttime dreams.

Ponder over a message sent
and where, oh, where your lifetime went.
And where it's going—ah, that's the best.
Tell about that, above the rest.
Record your darknesses and lights,
your loves, your depths, your fancy's flights

and lo, the moving finger writes!

—*by Alice Salerno, with permission*

Clearing Away & Setting the Foundation

chapter one

The Child

Congratulations on making a commitment and beginning to follow through. You are off to a great start.

The next step is to look back and explore childhood years, including beloved activities, foods, and people. You will also examine where some of your blocks to fitness may have originated. Let me start by sharing a little of my story.

As a child I lived *inside* my body, not outside of it looking back and criticizing it. My body was the vehicle that allowed me to run in the rain, build mud pies in the street, fight the neighbor boys (and win, I might add), fish with Dad, make cookies with Mom, sled, ski, ice skate, and many other wonderful family activities. It never occurred to me to look in the mirror. I was too busy being active. It felt as if the energy of the universe filled me and lifted me up like the kites we flew and lost as we watched them spiral out of control into the blue sky. Being active was about being a part of the fun, jumping into piles of leaves with my brother Mark, doing the Hustle with my brother John, camping with my brother Steve.

My father, a stocky Italian man with muscular arms and legs, was a football player in college. When I was a child, he was in good shape and an active hunter, fisherman, and camper. He took my brothers and me hiking, swimming, ice skating, skiing, camping, and sledding. He was competitive and viewed sports seriously, even as a coach for my brother's sports teams. I learned that if you were going to play sports, you had better be good, play hard, and win.

My mom was tall, lean, and graceful. She loved dancing and dreamt of being a Rockette before she married and had kids. When I was eight and started playing soccer, she said she wished she could have participated in sports when she was growing up. But girls weren't encouraged to play sports then, and in her small town, there were no sports teams for girls to join anyway. This angered and saddened me.

My father ate whatever he pleased, but my mom was more rigid about when, what, and how much to eat. I learned from them that eating was fun and cele-bratory—candy at Halloween, bobbing for apples at birthday parties, chips and soda when we went fishing—but also something to be controlled—no snacks before dinner, eat all your vegetables, don't eat too many sweets. As a child, I remember feeling starved between lunch and dinner, not allowed to snack, and wishing I had more control over when and what I ate. We were expected to clean our plates and eat foods we didn't like. I often secretly spit beets into my napkin.

Many happy family memories involved us gathering and eating during holi-days, birthdays, and other parties. But some sad times occurred then as well. One of the most painful memories during a family meal involved one of my brothers. He was slightly overweight, which bothered my dad. One night at dinner, Dad, who had an unpredictable temper, yelled at my fifteen-year-old brother, "You eat as if tomorrow will never come! No wonder you've gotten so fat!" His words stung. It was as though he had called my brother ugly and unacceptable in front of all of us. At eight years old, I was horrified, but now, more than twenty years later, I understand that Dad was afraid his son might be unsuccessful in life if he remained overweight.

My brother lost the excess weight as he got older and hasn't had a weight problem since. Ironically, my dad, because of poor eating and exercise habits, became overweight within a few years of this incident and remained that way. Unknowingly, as a child sitting at the dinner table, I began to develop attitudes and behaviors associated with food and weight that would continue for years.

Although I was athletic as a youngster, I was scared to death of pull-ups and climbing rope, which required upper body strength. Invariably, the gym teacher would force us to do these activities. I absolutely dreaded feeling that cold steel pull-up bar under my fingers and the stare of my fellow students on my back as they waited for me to give up so they could have their turn. I would tell myself, "Just get your chin above the bar once!" I would brace myself, squint, hold my breath and pull as hard as I could, but only move a fraction of an inch before dan-gling hopelessly from tiny arms. Dropping to my feet, I would walk past the gym teacher marking a big zero in her grade book and my classmates, some of whom were snickering at me.

As a result, I always thought I was hopelessly weak in my arms. What I've since learned is that genetically I don't have a lot of *power* in my arms, but I have *endurance*, a different kind of strength. I can train to increase both kinds of strength. I no longer have to feel ashamed or believe I am weak.

This chapter involves looking back at positive and negative childhood experiences associated with physical activity, diet, and body image. These memories will likely trigger all sorts of emotions: happiness, love, sadness, anger. Allow yourself to feel whatever comes up, without judgment. Doing this will free you to become and remain fit. It's like building a house. First, you must build a strong foundation, and in order to do that, sometimes you have to clear away old, outdated material; other times, you can simply restore the original.

Body/Self-Image

We all probably agree that it's much easier to love a child, especially when it's your own, than it is to love a teenager or an adult. We are more forgiving and accepting of children's imperfections; in fact, we often find these imperfections endearing. People love Anne Geddes's photographs of babies in all their wonderful shapes, sizes, and colors. Some babies have rolls of fat and chubby cheeks. Others are born premature with sheer skin that reveals every vein. Some are darker than night, while others are milky white. We buy cards, calendars, and books bearing photos of these marvelous babies. When was the last time you saw a book of photographs that celebrates the physical imperfections of teenagers or adults? By adolescence or adulthood, we no longer find our naturally varied body shapes to be adorable or even acceptable. We expect them to fit a certain predetermined mold.

Some of us have damaged ourselves physically, mentally, or spiritually in an effort to remake our bodies so others might love and accept us. If this is true for you, you may replay negative tapes in your mind while dismissing the positive, rejecting yourself, and withholding self-love. This book will help you see yourself as beautifully imperfect.

Physical Activity

Throughout this book, you will define which activities you enjoy. Why? Shouldn't you just force yourself to do whatever will get you the quickest results?

Adherence to a regular program of activity will increase if you enjoy it. And the longer you stick to a program, the better your chance for success.

What compels you to move may be different than what inspires someone else. Perhaps music would compel you to move even if you were in a body cast. Or maybe competition motivates you—no matter the sport, danger, or difficulty, if challenged, you'd compete. By identifying your hot buttons, you can work with your personality and preferences instead of against them.

Begin by listing your favorite physical activities in childhood. They do not have to be in any particular order of importance and they do not have to be organized sports or traditional exercises at all, although they could be. You could list Frisbee throwing, mud pie making, kite flying, fishing, dancing, chasing your dog, playing kickball. The activities can be ones you only did once or ones you did regularly.

Favorite Physical Activities in Childhood:

1.

2.

3.

4.

5.

Quickly think of one fitness/physical activity experience (or some other kind of success) in childhood that you're proud of. Maybe you caught the biggest fish. Or ran the second fastest time. Or beat up your neighborhood bully. Or did the high jump well. Share that experience here.

_____

_____

Now, close your eyes, and relive this experience. What was the weather like? How did it feel to be in your body? Who was with you? How did you know you did well? Did you receive praise, an award, or did you just feel good about it? Let yourself feel what it was like to be you at that moment. Jot down your memories and feelings in your journal.

Let's look at the other side of the coin—an embarrassing childhood experience involving appearance or ability in sports or fitness. Mine involved pull-ups in gym class, Janice's was being the heaviest person on the volleyball team, and Sally's had to do with feeling awkward.

What stands out most in your memory?

Did you avoid situations or people, shy away from those things that interested you because of shame, insecurity, fear?

Did you believe you were always going to be fat or thin, weak or strong, unlikable or popular?

To better understand your likes and dislikes, strengths and weaknesses, let's take a look at your family. Your parents may have had the greatest impact on you. Some of their influence might be obvious—perhaps you inherited your father's eyes and your mother's hair; other influences may be more obscure—perhaps you became outgoing or introverted or became overweight or underweight just like they were. They not only passed on physical genes but also attitudes, behaviors, and feelings, whether intending to or not.

Were your parents physically active during your childhood? What kind of attitudes did they have about fitness?

Were your siblings physically active? What did you learn either negatively or positively from this?

Were you an active child?

Food

Most of us probably have many pleasant memories associated with food. Life is too short not to have some simple pleasures. Which foods do you love and why? You may wonder why this is important. Most of us believe losing weight or body fat requires eliminating most foods we enjoy. This all-or-nothing thinking usually leads to trouble. Balance helps us adhere to a healthy lifestyle. If the routine is too strict or demanding, we'll either quit or not even begin. It may not be a great idea to buy five ice cream sandwiches from the ice cream truck because that was your favorite food as a kid, but eating one ice cream sandwich every now and then is fine. Food has probably played a big role in your life thus far and it probably always will. Deprivation leads to over-consumption later. The First Steps to Fitness program includes a Splurge Day once per week in which you can indulge in your favorite treats.

Quickly list foods from each meal that you particularly enjoyed in childhood:
Breakfast:
Lunch:
Dinner:
Special treat:
Snack:
Holidays:

These favorite foods may be ones you never allow yourself to have and thus could make potential rewards. When Ann created her list of rewards, she included one large, sweet, frosted Pop-Tart. Although she could've chosen anything, she chose a Pop-Tart because she had loved them as a child, but as an adult never allowed herself to have one.

Others may overeat these favorite childhood foods, perhaps trying to feed emotional hunger for comfort, happiness, a sense of youth. Do you tend to overeat any of the foods you listed?

The Chorus

The Chorus—these are the people who impacted your development. The Good News Chorus includes those who helped us feel good about ourselves. They were our champions. The term Bad News Chorus was coined in the book *Fitness Instinct* by Peg Jordan and refers to those who made us feel bad. We may find that some of the same people were in both our Good and Bad News choruses, which can be particularly confusing to a young person.

Who were your childhood champions? List them here, along with the positive feedback they gave you about yourself, your body, and/or appearance:

_____
_____
_____
_____
_____

Now turn to the Bad News Chorus. Several clients have painful childhood memories of being called names. Heidi was an overweight child, but not obese.

Everyone in her family was severely overweight, including her father. No one ate properly or exercised. Her legs were and still are the main focus of her insecurity. She described them as thick and undefined. Her father began calling her Tree Trunk Legs as a child and often forced her to diet and exercise.

His attempt at inspiring her to exercise made her feel more hopeless, fat, and unattractive. No amount of effort pleased him because he believed, just as she did, that she would grow up to be obese like everyone else. When she did diet, exercise, and lose weight, he responded, "Well, you'll just gain it back. You're gonna be just like your grandma." Her grandmother weighed four hundred pounds and could barely walk due to foot problems from the excess weight.

Thinking about these things made Heidi sad and angry, but remembering and identifying the roots of her insecurity allowed her to begin releasing them.

Not everyone has such painful memories, but most of my clients have some experiences that led to insecurities, unproductive habits or attitudes, or other problems with food, body image, and/or physical activity. As a child, did you have anyone in your Bad News Chorus? This chorus could include family members, friends, neighbors, acquaintances, classmates. Often, these people unintentionally hurt us. List them here along with the negative feedback they gave you about yourself, your body, and/or your appearance:

_____

_____

_____

_____

_____

Quickly list those things you wish you had experienced as a child or things you wish you'd done differently. (For example, not drop out of dance class, done at least one pull-up, stood up to the class bully who called you names, tried belly dancing.)

_____

_____

_____

_____

Are any of the items on the list ones you could someday accomplish, given the proper resources?

Exercises

1. Find a photo of yourself as a toddler. Which qualities do you find endearing? What emotions are bubbling up? Jot down what you're thinking and feeling as you look at the photo. In your journal, list as many positive things about this little child as you can, for example, "She has cute, oval eyes. They sparkle like she's really happy." Try to look at yourself in a nonjudgmental, loving way.

2. Find photos of yourself when you were approximately five or six years old, playing and moving around. What do you feel when you see yourself? Do you find yourself smiling when you look at these pictures? In your journal, describe your physical characteristics as a child. How did you compare to others your age? Were you shorter, taller, heavier, thinner than they were?

3. Draw a picture of yourself, a caricature that represents who you were as a child. If you were a happy child, you might draw a child with a huge grin on her face, or if you were silly, you might draw yourself as a clown. I drew myself as a tiny girl waving a big fist, which represented the contradiction between my little-girl frame and my big-boy attitude. How closely does your caricature reflect what you see in the photos? For example, if you drew a picture of yourself as a large child because that is how you thought of yourself, do the photos support this self-perception? Often some discrepancy exists between how we see ourselves and how we actually appear.

4. Describe how you felt as a child when you were active or when you were not. Also, in what ways did you participate in your fitness/sports development (i.e.: attend practices, try new things, take classes)? Explore these questions in your journal.

5. Find photos of your family at holiday get-togethers. As you gaze at the photos, jot down the thoughts and feelings that come to you. Were these

happy times? Did you learn to associate food/meals with family, fun, and celebration or with chaos, arguments, and isolation?

6. What kind of relationships did your family members have with food during your childhood? Were any of them over- or underweight? Were there rules about eating? Did you learn to use food for anything other than nutrition, such as killing emotions or time? What kinds of habits and attitudes regarding food did you pick up? Consider these questions in your journal.

7. Choose a meaningful word or phrase someone in your Good News Chorus said to you. Write it on a piece of paper and place it where you can read it every day. You could dress it up with a special font or add a drawing. You could frame it. Create a daily reminder that you are loved and lovable.

8. Choose someone from your Bad News Chorus and draw a caricature of him or her. You don't have to be an artist. It could be a funny sketch, such as a dragon with fire coming out of its nose or a wicked witch on her broom. Leave the drawing in your journal, burn it, cut it up into tiny pieces, call it a few names, throw darts at it, or do whatever helps you let go of some of the feelings you may have about the things this person said or did.

9. Write a letter to someone in your Bad News Chorus, not one that you will send, but one in which you express feelings that maybe you weren't able to express as a child.

10. Write a letter to yourself as a child, from you now. Tell yourself the things you needed to hear that you did not.

Check-In

1. How many days this week did you move for at least twenty minutes? Have you changed activities or tried new ones yet? Has it become easier or more enjoyable?

2. Which end-of-the chapter exercises were the most fun? The most difficult?

3. The most revealing?

4. Are you still committed to your fitness progress? Reread the contract you made with yourself.

chapter two

The Teen

You have faced and embraced childhood memories in chapter 1 and are now moving on to adolescence, one of the most illuminating and rewarding chapters in this book. For many, the teen years were a time of great change and excitement, but also disillusion and confusion. Some began to discover their strengths. Others experienced events that created feelings and behaviors that still haunt them today, making self-acceptance and self-improvement difficult. Although the particular experiences may have been different for each of us, the feelings were likely the same: excitement, insecurity, confidence, fear, pride, inadequacy, and more. For me, adolescence was a tumultuous time.

My dad still had the build of a brick house, but with an extra forty pounds around his midsection. He didn't take much time anymore to do those things he loved. His only consistent physical activity was gardening. Every six months or so, he'd feel shame for the shape he'd gotten into, so he would go for a run. Because he was out of shape, running was extremely difficult, and the agony would keep him from trying again for another six months. He was too macho to start by walking and, over time, build up to a run. He was five-feet, eleven-inches tall and weighed two hundred and twenty pounds. My mom didn't exercise at all until I was fifteen, when she started a jogging regimen.

The fat-free revolution hadn't hit yet, at least not in my house, and we followed the same routine: hot dogs, pot roast, hamburgers during the week, and pizza and donuts on the weekend. I had no idea what eating healthily meant. My dad ate whatever he wanted, especially sweets and fattening foods (not coincidentally, my favorites) and even tried to hide the extent of his bad habits. I often found empty candy bar and cigarette wrappers stuffed under the cushions in his truck. He denied they were his. Because my mom worked during the day, she couldn't make sure we ate right and often had to rely on one of us to make dinner. Since we didn't have much of a cooking repertoire, we made whatever was easiest but not necessarily the most nutritious.

After school, my brother Mark and I would eat graham crackers, chocolate milk, ice cream, and whatever else we could scrounge up while watching television. When I wasn't eating this way, I was living on chocolate, candies, cookies, shakes, and French fries with my friends. All adults had to do was tell us we couldn't have something and we'd find a way to get it. Our school wouldn't let students have gum, candy, or food in class, so if you had some and you shared, you were momentarily popular. Every day after school, we walked down the hill to the Hinky Dinky grocery store, played Ms. Pac-Man, and ate candy. To this day, I think of my girlfriends whenever I see a bag of Jolly Ranchers.

My brothers were all active in sports, and their involvement motivated me to play. I have many proud memories of watching them hit the ball, shoot the hoop, throw a pass, score a goal. I wanted to be just like them.

My friends were athletic, coordinated, and interested in playing sports or being on the drill team. We did things together such as go out for track in the ninth grade. We were all competitive, but we acted as a team no matter what sport we were playing.

My parents supported my brothers and my involvement in sports, taking us to games, watching us play, cheering us on; however, my dad took the game too seriously sometimes, which caused hurt feelings. When I was thirteen, he yelled at me after a soccer game. He said that I should've followed the coach until he let me back in the game and should've been more aggressive on the field. All I could think about was that my dad had never played soccer in his life, so he had no right to criticize me. But I didn't say a word. Scared of him, I bottled the anger inside and secretly wished he would never come to another game. After his criticism, I began to question my soccer ability.

My dad never did attend another game. Several months after this experience, he died suddenly from a blood clot that formed after a surgery. The clot moved to his heart, growing to the size of a baseball, and cut off air and blood flow. The doctors told us after Dad died that the clot most likely would not have formed if he had exercised, eaten right, and not smoked.

I was angry at my dad when he died. As a rebellious, confused teenager, I had been having trouble getting along with him. He seemed to want me to act like a lady when up to that point my tomboyish, risk-taking nature had pleased him.

Once I began to develop physically, wear makeup, and hang around with boys, he tried to protect me, but I perceived this as an attempt to control me. I would not be controlled. After his death, I felt guilty that I had pushed him away and sad that he and I wouldn't have the chance to work out our differences.

I spent the next year rebelling—partying with friends, skipping church, and slacking off in school. I experienced more loss when my last brother moved away, my mom sold the house we had lived in as a family, and my then-boyfriend went to college. I spent a lot of time alone thinking about everything and fell into a horrible depression. Subconsciously, I began to punish myself for everything I thought I'd done wrong and began to try to improve myself. Within two years, I went from a party girl to a loner obsessed with physical, scholastic, and religious perfection.

Overexercising by running, dancing, playing soccer, and severely restricting my diet, I lost weight, not to make myself attractive, but to punish myself and to feel some control over my life. As I lost more and more weight, people began to worry. I didn't care. Their comments only fueled my deepening shame about my body and myself. I saw no way out of my feelings and therefore no way out of my behaviors. Afraid of how much it would hurt, I couldn't tell anyone how I felt, sure no one would understand.

I lost more than 25 percent of my body weight, my breasts disappeared, my menstrual cycle stopped for four years, my clothes hung on me, a light down grew on my sallow skin, and my thick hair began to fall out. Still, I didn't care what happened to me. In some way, I enjoyed destroying myself. I had no mercy because I had no love for myself. Without knowing it, I had developed anorexia.

This continued until my drive for perfection nearly killed me. Because I could never, never be good enough, I felt worse about myself after trying so hard and, in my eyes, failing. Having isolated myself from others, I felt more alone. I couldn't allow anyone to love me because I wasn't "perfect" and thus not worthy of love.

I realize now that feeling abandoned after Dad died, I completely abandoned myself. I was no longer the happy-go-lucky, funny, excited person I had been but had become someone trying to fit into a box I thought everyone, including God, wanted me to fit into. Once in the box, I wanted to die, and in effect already had.

Not until I was an adult did I fully examine my feelings about exercise, diet, and body image, and I found many had their roots in my unhealthy adolescence.

However minor or major, painful issues I thought I had left behind were blocking my progress.

Much of what I learned growing up, I picked up unknowingly:

1. Exercise is something you don't want to do because it is painful.
2. Exercise is different from sports and other activities because it isn't fun.
3. Sports and enjoyable fitness activities are for kids. Adults shouldn't take time to do these things.
4. If you play sports, you should win.
5. Adults aren't expected to stay in good shape.
6. Getting out of shape as you get older is inevitable.
7. Exercise is something you *should* do.
8. Go to extremes—don't exercise or eat right at all, or do it too much.
9. If you don't eat right and exercise, you will die before your time.

Do any of these sound familiar?

After reading that I had been anorexic, one client, Rita, told me she thought, "Oh, no. Not another one of them." She couldn't relate to someone who didn't eat because her problem was overeating. However, like me, she had experienced situations growing up that affected her body image, self-esteem, and behavior patterns. How these experiences manifest themselves—whether through over- or undereating or over- or underexercising—doesn't matter. The solution is still the same. Uncover the positive. Discover and discard the negative. And build a solid foundation.

Physical Fitness

Now, let's talk about the physical activities you enjoyed as a teen. One client, Jenny, radiated with pride when she told me how in shape she had been in high school. She had been a cheerleader, volleyball player, and swimmer. Since then, she had struggled with her weight, especially after giving birth to two children. When she came to me, she was eighty pounds overweight. I asked her to describe the activities she used to do and how she looked and felt doing them. She had nearly forgotten the pride, confidence, and energy she had felt. The idea of regaining that feeling excited and frightened her, but day by day she worked on herself, inside and out. She began to do some of those activities she once loved such as dancing, skating, hiking, and swimming. Gradually, she shed weight and regained confidence.

Fill in the chart below with your favorite physical activities in adolescence. Kissing doesn't count! The activities needn't be in any particular order of importance and don't necessarily have to be organized sports or traditional exercises. You could list soccer, softball, gardening, golfing, fishing, horseback riding, skating, or jumping rope.

Favorite Physical Activities in Adolescence:

1.
2.
3.
4.
5.

Now categorize each activity, choosing from the list below. For example, let's say you chose soccer. Looking over the list, you would probably select the words competitive, fast-paced, and team activity to describe this sport. Then, you would write these three descriptions next to soccer. Do this for each activity on your list.

Categories:

1. Competitive
2. Noncompetitive
3. Fast-paced
4. Moderate-paced
5. Slow-paced
6. Team activity
7. Solitary activity

Did you see a pattern with the kinds of activities you chose? Did they all have similar descriptions? Or were they different? What categories of activity did you prefer? Were any of your choices the same as your childhood favorites?

Now let's talk about how your parents and family affected your views on fitness. Though you probably thought you were old enough to make up your mind about everything, your parents/family were still leading by example. What kind of example did your parents set?

- During your teen years, what was the state of their health? Their appearance?
- Did they exercise? If so, were they active because they enjoyed it or because they knew they "should"?
- Did you follow in their footsteps?
- Do you remember them saying anything derogatory about their own or each other's bodies? If so, how did this make you feel?
- Did you and your siblings play together as teens?
- Were you jealous of each other's abilities, or did you support each other?
- Did you want to be like them?
- Did your parents support any physical activities you wanted to pursue? How?
- Was their "help" helpful or not?
- Did anything happen that made you feel more secure or less secure about your abilities?

Our peers impacted our thoughts and behaviors. They were sometimes even more influential in our development than our family, much to our parents' chagrin. We often emulated our friends to fit in.

Some clients did not have athletic friends like I had in adolescence. These clients may have wanted to play sports and be active, but they didn't have the courage to do it alone and their friends wouldn't do it with them. Naturally, to fit in, they chose to do what their friends did.

- Did you have friends who encouraged you to be active?
- Did you play sports or do other fitness activities together?
- Did you attract people who were just like you? Or did you change yourself to be like them?
- Did you compete with your friends or work as a team?

As teens, we often compared ourselves negatively with our peers. A client, Sally, told me that she had always felt less coordinated and more awkward than her friends and still feels that way about herself. She didn't appear ungraceful to me. It was a *feeling* of awkwardness, not a reality. Another client, Kim, also compared herself to her peers. She was heavier than most of them and was ashamed of her body. She didn't risk getting involved in physical activities that may have embarrassed her even more.

- How did your physical abilities compare with your peers'?
- Did you think they were better, worse, or the same as you?
- If you felt they were better, did you end up quitting or trying even harder?
- What do you see now that you couldn't see then?

Diet

Perhaps your diet, like mine, took a nosedive in your teen years. You may have had more freedom to do what you wanted, which may have included eating foods that weren't always good for you. You may have begun to ignore or even rebel against any dietary controls your parents tried to establish. Or you may have begun learning about healthy eating and developed an interest in cooking.

- Did the family diet change from your childhood to your adolescence?
- What kind of diet did your parents have?
- Was there one set of standards for you and one for them?
- Did you eat out a lot or have home-cooked meals?
- Did you learn to cook, and, if so, what kinds of foods?

List the most common foods you ate with your family:

_____

_____

_____

_____

Are these foods you eat now? Many of us ate whatever our friends ate just to be cool. Maybe your parents told you fruits and vegetables were good for you, and since doing anything your parents said was considered uncool, you did the opposite and ate junk food.

- What did you eat with your friends?
- Did you consider junk food to be fun?

- Did you go to other people's houses for their food or did they come to yours?

List the foods you and your friends thought were the best:

_____

_____

_____

_____

Are they still a part of your diet? The hormonal changes of puberty may have influenced your eating patterns and choices even without your realizing it. You may have begun to crave certain foods, eat more, put on weight, have mood swings. These changes and the reactions of those around you may have frightened you, especially if you didn't understand these changes as natural and necessary to becoming a physically mature woman.

Some reacted to changes in their bodies by trying to control them through diet and exercise. Did you and/or your friends diet? Did you fear calories or getting fat? Did you develop an eating disorder?

Body Image

As a child, you might not have spent much time preening in front of a mirror or worrying about what others thought of your appearance. Adolescence changed this for some. Suddenly, they wanted boys to find them attractive. They became willing to do whatever necessary to look a certain way. Parents may have begun to worry that if their child didn't look good, she wouldn't have friends or be successful. Conditions of love and acceptance may have laid the foundation for a negative body image.

- When did you first begin to care about your attractiveness?
- Who did you use as a measuring stick? Models? Friends? Actresses? Sisters?
- What did you like the most about your appearance when you were a teenager?

Find photos of yourself in junior high and/or high school. List three or more things you liked about your physical appearance then.

_____

_____

_____

_____

_____

Also, jot down three or more personal attributes (besides physical ones) that you liked about yourself, such as intelligence, sense of humor, creativity.

_____

_____

_____

_____

_____

What did you like least about your appearance?

_____

_____

_____

What did you try to change?

_____

_____

_____

Some of us tried all kinds of things to be attractive and often ended up looking worse for the effort. My hair literally took up almost the entire square of my eighth grade yearbook picture. Why? Because I was trying to feather it back like all my friends did. However, their hair was thin and fine and feathered back flat and soft, while mine was thick and curly and stuck out three inches from my head.

Body image became a problem for some of us when we suddenly had hips, more body fat, and breasts.

- How old were you when you began going through puberty?
- If you were one of the first or last girls to go through it, how did this impact you?
- What kind of physical transformation did you undergo?
- How did your family react to the changes you were going through physically and emotionally?
- Did they make it easier or more difficult to deal with these changes?

The Chorus

It can be easier to dwell on criticism than on compliments. Perhaps somewhere along the way we were taught it was conceited to have pride about our bodies or anything else. Positive attention may have been embarrassing, so we avoided these situations. The negative remained in our heads like bells ringing over and over again, whereas the positive was buried and forgotten. Is this true for you?

Think back to compliments you were given about your appearance or abilities in junior high and high school. Revel in these memories for a while. List these nice things you remember hearing and watch how your mind tries to minimize and negate them. Keep writing anyway.

_____

_____

_____

_____

_____

_____

On the flip side, who made up your Bad News Chorus in adolescence?

Let me tell you about my friend Alice. Her father was an overachiever, an accomplished businessman who wanted her to be successful too. He felt she needed to improve her appearance. Like him, she had problems with her weight, only he dieted and exercised to "improve" himself while she did not. The more he tried to convince her to lose weight, exercise, eat right, and become as concerned about her appearance as he was, the angrier and more hurt she became.

She interpreted his "help" as evidence that he didn't love her, that he just wanted to control her and make her be like him. Feeling unlovable, she became depressed. The more depressed she became, the more she ate. Unable to admit to her dad that she was angry and hurt, she couldn't let go of her negative self-image and behaviors.

Did you ever feel that love from others was conditional based upon how you looked? If so, did you try to meet or exceed expectations? Or did you rebel and not try at all?

Another client, Linda, realized as she worked through this section of the book that her weight problem began at age sixteen, when she had to give up sports and cheerleading so she could work after school. A year later, still working, she was allowed to play one sport and chose volleyball. The coaches noticed she had gained fifteen to twenty pounds and insisted she lose weight, even though she was five-feet four-inches tall and a normal 130 pounds. They required her to bring a bag lunch instead of allowing her to eat pizza or burgers with the rest of the team after games. She recalled feeling flattered by her coaches' attention but also embarrassed for being singled out as "fat." Ever since, she thought of herself as fat and struggled with her weight.

Now that you've examined your physical activity, diet, and body image in childhood and adolescence, perhaps you have seen how your past has affected your fitness today and have begun to free yourself from negative patterns that have stood in your way. As you move from studying adolescence to examining your present life, consider these questions:

- What insecurities did you take with you from adolescence to adulthood?
- What hopes and dreams?
- Are these still with you today?

Exercises

1. What, approximately, was your weight, height, and clothing size when you were sixteen? How did you feel about yourself then?

2. Describe in your journal what you and your friends considered attractive. Name people (friends, movie stars, models) you thought fit the bill. How did you compare? Were you thinner, bigger, or the same size as these role models? Were your expectations realistic?

3. Take one or more of the compliments you received in adolescence and jot them on a piece of paper. Attach it to a mirror or the front of your journal or the refrigerator, somewhere where you will read it every day.

4. Draw four columns lengthwise on a piece of paper. In the first column, list everyone in your Bad News Chorus during adolescence, all those who said or did harmful things to you. In the second column, write what they said or did. In the third, describe your corresponding feelings as well as you can remember. In the fourth, record your initial reactions to each event (withdrawing, getting angry, fighting) and also any delayed reactions (dieting, working out, feeling sorry for yourself, overeating, falling into a depression, shrugging it off).

5. After filling them all in, review the third and fourth columns. Do you see a pattern in your emotions and reactions?
• Did you tend to overeat every time someone put you down?
• Did you try to please everyone and live up to unrealistic expectations?
• Did you tell yourself you didn't care, seem unaffected by others' criticism?
• What part, through your reactions, did you play in your own self-esteem/body image development?

Take any of the questions posed earlier in this chapter and explore it in depth in your journal.

Check-In

1. How many days this week did you move for at least twenty minutes? Have you changed activities or tried new ones yet? Has it become easier

or more enjoyable?

2. How many of the exercises at the end of the chapter have you been able to do? Which ones have been the most fun? The most difficult? The most revealing?

3. Reread your Commitment Contract. Are you remaining committed? Why or why not?

chapter three

The Adult

You've covered a lot of ground exploring childhood and adolescence. You've uncovered some influences that may have set you up for your present circumstances. Now you'll define your present outlook and behaviors. If you don't, it will be like trying to manage a store without knowing how many products you have to sell and how much you need to order. You'll do a personal inventory of your exercise, diet, and body image as an adult. This will allow you to move beyond what you have *believed* to be true to what *is* true. You can begin to shape your life into what you *want* instead of what you *do not* want.

When we become adults, we're so much wiser, right? Maybe in some areas, but maybe *not* in others. As I got older, I got better at pretending to be happy and having it all together. Every year, I became more adept at hiding myself from others as well as from myself, just as I hid under baggy clothes.

Entering adulthood, I carried with me the same obsession with calories and exercise I had as an adolescent. I was still afflicted with what I call mental anorexia. Because I was no longer physically anorexic, I thought my problems were solved. However, since I had not dealt with the emotions and thoughts that had supported my tendency toward self-destruction, I still had problems. I had simply gained enough weight so no one would worry about me, and so I could continue in denial.

My obsessive thought patterns and insecurities made relationships with others difficult. I became very shy. I might have stayed stuck forever if it hadn't been for some loving, honest people who saw past my "disguise" as a well-adjusted individual and found ways to help me.

Lauren, a family friend, recognized that I didn't have it all together as much as I wanted everyone to believe. She had also been anorexic and understood how the negative thoughts and feelings could linger for years, despite outward appearance. She had been there, but she had worked on herself both outwardly and inwardly. She told me about her past struggles and the path she took to freedom. Her honesty helped me to take another look at my experiences and share them with her.

From her and other friends, I learned some important, life-changing lessons. The most important realization was that I had allowed other people—their opinions, words, and actions—to have too much power over me. I realized I was not a victim unless I allowed myself to be. I possessed the power to be an active participant in my life and in finding solutions to my problems. I could begin a new life if I continued to be honest and if I learned how to be loving and responsible.

No matter how much a person tries to love another, she will always disappoint the loved one in some ways because she is human. It's impossible for anyone to love 100 percent unconditionally all the time. I had to quit expecting this from my own loved ones. Instead of relying on other people to reinforce my self-image, Lauren suggested that through prayer and meditation I find a source of unconditional love. She recommended I list all of my positive attributes besides physical ones to help me see myself as more than just a body. She and others helped me understand than I had rejected myself but I didn't have to do that anymore. Honesty and faith were my keys to a new life.

That was twelve years ago. Since then I have been working through the issues that led me to repeat self-defeating patterns with exercise and diet. Working out is no longer a self-punishing, solitary activity for me. It has become an enjoyable part of my life to share with clients, friends, and family. I taught my mother the First Steps to Fitness weight and aerobic workout. She's followed it, has had good results, and she loves it. She tells me she's getting "buff" and even flexes her biceps for people. My brothers continue to be active in sports and other activities they enjoy. My husband plays basketball, runs occasionally, and has also begun lifting weights with me. We enjoy walking, bike riding, running, roller blading, and dancing together. I'm fortunate to have such good examples and wonderful people to share these things with me.

I love food. Is that a surprise, coming from an ex-anorexic? Well, I always have and always will love food. For me, as for most anorexics, not eating was about control, willpower, and self-deprivation. That's no way to live. Eating can be a healthy source of fun, sharing, and pleasant memories. My husband and I both appreciate good food. One of our hobbies is finding great gourmet restaurants and sharing these places with friends and family. During the week, we have low-fat, balanced meals, but on weekends we go out to our favorite places.

It's much easier to eat healthfully when those around you do the same. But let's face it, most people don't eat this way. However, it's possible to eat right even when you're surrounded by people who don't. It is a test of the saying, "to thine own self be true." Not everyone is health-conscious or supportive. Often when I'm eating with such people they try to pressure me into eating foods they eat—hamburgers, fries, baked goods—which are foods I do enjoy occasionally. If I am true to myself, I don't eat these things in order to fit in, so others don't think I'm weird or compulsive. To be true to myself I eat, exercise, and do those things that make me feel good, regardless of what others around me are doing. My husband also enjoys a healthy diet, but if he didn't, I still would because it makes *me* feel good and because then I don't have to work harder to keep those treats from settling on my thighs.

Balancing exercise and healthy eating has become easier for me because my definition of an attractive woman has changed. It's easier not to starve myself or feel guilty about eating since I no longer think being rail-thin is attractive. Instead, shapely curves and toned muscles look good. I can't be shapely and toned if I don't eat and if I don't lift weights. Females were meant to have curves.

I keep a balanced perspective by reminding myself that my physical life is only temporary. I certainly don't ignore my body, but it is not my primary focus either. And most importantly, I am grateful for what I have. I have found a direction for my life in sharing this balanced perspective with clients and in writing about my experiences to help others.

Body Image

For some of you, the hardest part of this program will be coming up with what you *like* about your body as an adult. You might catch yourself falling prey to reverse pride. Thinking you're worse than you are can be as detrimental as being too prideful. Most likely you're somewhere in the middle, not perfect but certainly not horrible. My clients have learned to share the nice things they think about their bodies. Diana, for instance, told me that she used to stop traffic with her legs. Mary reflected that she was once a size four and looked good in sexy, tight-fitting clothes. Carole said that she had been in phenomenal physical shape in college. Even though she hadn't been thin, she had *felt attractive*.

Beside each part of the body listed below, quickly jot down the first thought that comes to your mind.

My face _____

My hair _____

My chest _____

My back _____

My arms _____

My abdomen _____

My butt _____

My thighs _____

My inner thighs _____

My outer thighs _____

My calves _____

After answering, read over your responses and classify them as critical, positive, or neutral. Critical would be anything that points out flaws or faults. Positive would be pointing out what is good. Neutral would be a nonjudgmental response such as *OK* or *acceptable* as a response to, for example, *my abdomen*. Did you have more negative than positive responses?

You might answer, "I say critical things about myself because I'm fat!" or "I'm not being critical, I'm being honest!" Honesty is good, but so is accepting that there's more to you than just appearance. For example, let's say you wrote that your arms are flabby when you could have written functional, useful, or healthy. Why judge your body parts by appearance instead of their function or health? We never think, "Gosh, that cellulite on my bottom may come in handy if there's ever a famine or I get really sick and can't eat." No, we think, "Gosh, that cellulite looks gross!" We've been conditioned to think about our bodies as *objects* instead of as *amazingly complex temples* that house our thoughts, feelings, and dreams.

Return to the list above and add at least one positive statement to what you have already written. For example, let's say the first thought that came into your mind when you read *my legs* was the word *chubby*. Now, go back and add something positive about them such as *strong* or *useful*.

We judge our bodies as good, bad, neutral, and often quit there, judging our bodies as ourselves. As a result, we see ourselves as good, bad, or neutral. In other words, our body image can often determine our entire self-image. Isn't that sad? Isn't that putting us all into little boxes that only fitness can bring us out of? That's a lot of pressure to put on ourselves—to remold our bodies into what society currently considers attractive. How many of us think, "I may not be gorgeous or have the perfect body according to today's standards, but I *am* strong, smart, biologically amazing, and worthwhile"?

Striving for beauty can hold us back from developing in other areas. A friend confided that if she could make herself beautiful—clear skin, toned body, perfect hair—then she'd be happy. When I asked what she would do once she had achieved this beauty, she said, "I'd get on with my life," spending more energy on favorite hobbies and searching for a career she loved. Ironically, she was already beautiful.

Roughly a third of my clients come to me in good shape with healthy body fat percentages and weight ranges. Why do they seek personal training? Generally, as we begin, they complain about some aspect of their bodies—lack of tone, too much cellulite, or too wide here or there. They often call themselves fat when they aren't.

Angie was one of these clients. She was not overweight, but her mother and sister were and she was afraid she would become like them. She admitted she had always had to work hard to maintain her slim physique. Her family loved eating and so did she. Fear of becoming fat made her feel as if she already was, and her fear led her to eat more than she intended to, take long breaks from exercise, and become depressed and frustrated. Since it was her negative body image creating this fear, her body image was keeping her stuck.

Why do so many of us think we're worse than we really are? Why are we so hard on ourselves? There are many reasons, but one has to do with what we see every day in magazines and on TV.

Lisa wanted to look like the women in body-building magazines who have less than 10 percent body fat. Slim and fit, she only had 18 percent body fat. Aspiring for greater fitness is fine, no matter what level you have already attained. Problems begin when you see yourself as fat when you aren't, or see yourself in any way inaccurately and/or negatively. Although Lisa didn't actually call herself fat when we were together, she did make comments that revealed her unhappiness with her physique as compared to the women in the magazines.

Though other clients complimented Lisa's nice physique, she disliked her arms because they weren't muscular enough, and her legs because they were too big and undefined. This isn't what I, or others in the gym, saw when we looked at her. Her negative self-perception motivated her to come to the gym three times a week and lift weights for a while, but after a couple of months, when she still didn't look like the women in the magazines, she quit coming.

Initially, negative body image can act as a catalyst for fitness. However, this kind of motivation doesn't work in the long term, because any negative motivation eventually turns on itself.

Have you ever worked for a boss who tried to motivate you by pointing out everything you did wrong and saying little or nothing about what you did right? You may have first tried to please him/her, but after repeatedly doing your best without positive feedback, you begin to lose hope. If, for all your hard work, someone persists in pointing out your imperfections, however minor, your motivation eventually fades. How many times will you try to please before you realize you'll never live up to expectations? You may continue to work with fear and anxiety as motivation, or you may become angry and resentful and start skipping work or talking about your boss behind his/her back, or taking longer breaks than you should.

Without positive reinforcement and motivation, we rebel or give up. The same is true with fitness. However, here you are your own boss. If the boss is too lax, nothing gets done. If too demanding, negativity takes over. In order to progress, you'll need to hold yourself accountable for your actions and have an accurate and forgiving body image.

The Chorus

Hopefully, there have been people in your adult life who have been your champions, who love you as you are, support you, and show that they believe in you. Think back to coworkers, family, friends, and even strangers. What *nice* things have people said to you in adulthood about the way you look, about who you are and/or about what you do? As fast as you can, jot these down in the spaces provided. You don't have to agree with what they said. In fact, you probably don't, but that doesn't matter right now. It's not necessary to recall the details of who said what or when, just what was said in general. Whatever you can remember, put it down.

_____

_____

_____

_____

Now, look back at your Good News Chorus in chapters 1 and 2.
- Are some chorus members on all three lists?
- Have you received similar feedback in each stage of life?
- Can you accept compliments? Or do you suffer from reverse pride that tells you you're worse than you are?
- Do you need to improve your picture of yourself?

Often a significant other will say something nice about how we look and we automatically assume they want something from us or simply want us to stop complaining. Has this ever happened to you? If so, perhaps you couldn't accept the words because you couldn't accept yourself. As you work through this book, you will find that you are better able to receive compliments and accept your body.

Do others support your wish to be more physically fit? Or do they put obstacles in your way, such as their poor attitudes, negativity, or neediness? Janet, a client, is a good example of someone who experienced and overcame such obstacles. Her husband was out of shape and hadn't exercised for years. He constantly complained about her going to the gym two nights a week, leaving him with their children. She almost let his complaints derail her until she and I discussed the situation. She realized that it wasn't his complaints that were tempting her to quit, but her guilt about being away from her kids. The solution was to talk to her husband about how important it was for her health and self-esteem to lose her pregnancy weight. She stressed to him that she was serious about this commitment.

She knew her kids would benefit by having a mom who was happier with herself. She also wanted to provide a healthier example for her five-year-old daughter, who was already overweight for her age.

Ironically, what Janet feared would pull her family apart when she first began working out actually brought them closer together. Her daughter became her greatest supporter, cheering her on when she lost inches and fit into smaller clothes. She begged her mom to let her go to the gym with her and danced alongside her at home while Janet did exercise videos. Her husband also developed an enthusiasm for exercising and eating right. They began working out as a family, going on bike rides, roller blading, hiking, and began preparing healthy meals together. If Janet had allowed her husband's initial resistance to dissuade her, she wouldn't have reaped these rewards.

Sometimes people attempt to be supportive only to wind up hurting our feelings. Below are two extreme examples.

One of my clients received a box of diet pills from her husband for Valentine's Day. When she opened the gift, she started crying and her husband apparently had no idea why. He knew she wanted to lose weight and thought she'd appreciate his help. After talking it out, he understood she had interpreted his gift as criticism.

On several occasions at the gym, I overheard a man talking to his wife as they worked out together. He insisted she would have the body she wanted if she just did exactly as he said without question. As he griped at her for resting too long or for not lifting enough weight, she bowed her head in silence. Eventually, they stopped coming to the gym together.

Although people may resist our efforts to improve ourselves or may inadvertently hurt our feelings, we don't have to let them control our behavior. We make the choice.

Diet

Quickly list foods from each meal that you particularly enjoy as an adult:
Breakfast:
Lunch:
Dinner:
Special treat:
Snack:
Holidays:

Glance over the foods. How many have similar qualities such as sweet or salty, fatty or spicy?

Compare your favorites now to ones you chose in childhood and adolescence. Have they changed? Or do you continue to favor the same kinds of foods?

I found that most of my favorites are sweet. Why is this important? I knew that sweets can be my downfall, but I didn't realize the extent to which this was true, or that it had been a pattern since childhood. You probably have natural tendencies toward certain foods just as you do toward physical activities. You shouldn't try to change your natural tendencies, but instead learn to balance them with other foods you need (with one day to splurge, of course) and with activities that suit you now.

- How do you use food? Your favorite foods may be ones you have used or still use as a reward or for comfort. They may also be a habit or ritual.
- Do you eat because you're hungry, or when you're sad, stressed, or bored?
- If you occasionally eat for emotional reasons, what are those?
- Which emotions trigger eating? Knowing these things about yourself will allow you to be watchful and modify your reactions.

Another client, Jessica, was trying to lose weight, but every weekend when she and her family went to the movies, she had a tub of buttered popcorn. She couldn't imagine the ritual of family day at the movies without the buttery smell, crunching sound, and salty taste of popcorn. She and I discussed alternatives such as bringing homemade, lower-fat popcorn with her to the movies. She tried doing this. Supplied with her healthier alternative, she didn't feel physically or emotionally deprived. And she didn't have any guilt. She could lose weight without having to forfeit the fun associated with food.

Is it possible to eat a healthy diet if everyone else in your household or work environment is eating unhealthy food? Passing up a plate of cookies and reaching for an apple instead is difficult. Preparing cookies for family, classmates, or coworkers and not eating some yourself is nearly impossible. Changing to a low-fat diet when your husband prefers full-fat foods is challenging. How can you do it? How much resistance would there be to changing the whole family's diet? Before you try it, though, identify your family's current diet habits and attitudes.

List your family's favorite foods:
1.
2.
3.
4.
5.

How many of these foods are also your favorites? How many of these are healthy? It's tough to look at the part we've played in developing poor eating habits in our children. In the United States, the incidence of obesity among children has more than doubled in the last thirty years. They are following their adult role models.

Once you've decided to eat wisely, no matter what others around you choose to do, others often become supportive. Sometimes they even begin eating the same foods too, without complaint. This new behavior can become natural for the whole family, in spite of their initial resistance.

Physical Activity

Being an adult probably involves having to do way too many things you would prefer not to do. Why add to the list when you don't have to? Sometimes you may feel as if you have no choice but to do exercises you dislike. In this chapter, you'll discover why you feel this way and how to become open to more desirable choices.

One of the first questions I ask new clients is what kind of exercises they have done in the past *that they enjoyed*. Most come up with at least one. Why would I put them on a bike when they've just told me they hate bicycling but love walking? I get them walking and both our jobs are easier.

You may answer, "Yeah, but what I like to do doesn't really count as 'exercise,'" or "I can burn calories faster by running instead of walking, even though I love to walk." But remember, if you're doing something you love, you'll do it longer and more often and thus burn more calories while doing what makes you feel good. At the end of a bad day or when you're facing one, do an exercise you love, instead of one you think you should do. You'll feel refreshed as a result.

Favorite Physical Activities in Adulthood:

1.
2.
3.
4.
5.

Did you have difficulty coming up with activities or did you have trouble narrowing it down? Review your Favorite Activities lists from chapters 1 and 2 and compare them to the list above. Put a star next to your adult favorites that you also chose for childhood and adolescence.

Next to each item on the list, write the approximate month or year you last enjoyed that activity. You may discover you haven't done some of them in a long time.

Now categorize your favorite activities in adulthood just as you did in chapter 2 by choosing from the list below:

• Competitive
• Noncompetitive
• Fast-paced
• Moderate-paced
• Slow-paced
• Team activity
• Solitary activity

Between chapters 2 and 3, which three categories did you choose the most? Jot them down here:

_____
_____
_____
_____

These three categories describe your fitness personality, what naturally appeals to you in sports and other forms of movement. Jot down other activities that fit the same description—ones you've never done, ones you don't think you can do, or ones you're scared of trying. List the first activities that come to mind.

1.
2.
3.
4.
5.

As we grew older, many of us stopped doing what we used to do to stay in shape. We may have gained weight, lost motivation, gotten injured, or become too busy. Maybe we think that if we can't participate in the sports we love, then there's nothing else we want to do. Maybe it isn't so much the sport itself, but some other aspect of it such as the team spirit, excitement, or challenge that we love. By identifying why these particular activities appeal to us, perhaps we can find alternatives we can equally enjoy.

Cathy was on a gymnastics team in high school and college and loved it. When she began training with me, she was in her late thirties, worked forty-plus hours a week, and was somewhat out of shape. Although she would have loved to join a gymnastics team, it wasn't practical. After talking about her gymnastics memories, she discovered she missed the camaraderie and teamwork more than the sport itself. She realized she was more likely to continue exercising if she did so with friends and if they worked toward a common goal such as finishing a mini-triathlon together.

You probably have some fitness successes as an adult that you'd benefit from remembering, such as finishing a race, participating in an event, reaching a goal, or learning a new sport. Success isn't always about appearance. It can be measured in happiness, strength, commitment, consistency, and pride. The client in my next story experienced all of these.

When Natalie began working out, she weighed two hundred pounds and was about fifty pounds overweight. After six months of doing the First Steps to Fitness program, she had lost twenty-five pounds, 6 percent of her body fat, and had gained significant strength. Recently, she was in the gym waiting for a fit young man to finish with the leg press machine. He was lifting 290 pounds. When he saw Natalie was going to use the machine next, he began to take the weight off. When she told him to stop—290 pounds was the weight she warmed up with—

his jaw dropped. He watched her do the leg press, but when she began adding more weight, he left, shaking his head. He didn't know that she increased the weight to 450 pounds, which was quite an improvement over the 160 pounds she pressed when she first started training.

Write about your successes here:

_____

_____

_____

_____

_____

_____

Exercises

1. Find the most recent photo of yourself. What do you like about yourself? Explore this in your notebook.

2. This next exercise demonstrates how we learn through visual stimulus even without our conscious awareness. Gather several magazines. Leaf through the pages and cut out every picture of a woman that you come across. Count the total number of women you found and write down this number. Then count the number of the women in the photos who you would classify as thin. Write this number down. Divide the number of thin women by the total number of women to get the percentage of those who are thin. Next, count how many of the thin women are also shown to be successful—smiling, wealthy, happy, with the man of their dreams. Is there apparently a correlation between thinness and success? Describe your observations in your journal.

3. Think of yourself as your body's fitness boss. What kind of boss have you been? Kind, but stern? Unbending? Too lax? Are you happy under this kind of leadership? If not, what kind of boss would you like to be?

4. How do others around you seem to feel about their bodies? What do they say about themselves? List the people you spend the most time with in a

week. Then, next to their names, rate them with a number between one and ten that represents how you think they perceive their bodies. A one represents an extremely negative body image, and a ten represents a very positive body image. How many seem to feel good about their bodies? How do you think they would rate your body image?

5. What personal attributes do you need to accept but cannot? Perhaps you have been told you have nice legs but have never accepted the compliment. Maybe you have a great sense of humor but don't give yourself credit for it. List the positive attributes most difficult to accept and post the list where you can read it daily.

6. List those who make up your Bad News Chorus in adulthood. How many were also in your childhood or adolescent Bad News Chorus? Do you agree or disagree with criticisms given to you as an adult? How have these comments made you feel and how have you reacted? For example, have you dieted, exercised, popped diet pills, or somehow altered your life to win others' approval? Or have you given up, deciding you could never measure up?

7. Name the people in your life (family, friends, coworkers) who support your desire to be fit. Then on the next page, list those who are unsupportive. Beside the names on each list, jot down the kinds of support they are or are not providing you:
    • **Operational:** watching the kids so you can go to the gym, preparing healthy meals, making it easier for you to leave work or home so you can work out
    • **Emotional:** listening, not judging, giving good advice based on their own experiences
    • **Motivational:** encouraging you to do what you want to do, telling you how well you're doing, complimenting you
    • **Financial:** supporting your desire to purchase fitness equipment, services, healthy food, supplements, or whatever other products you need

  • **Personal:** working out with you, meeting you at the gym, working through this book as well, or in some way traveling on the fitness path with you

8. Now, glance over your Supportive versus Non-Supportive lists. Which list has more names?
    • What kind of support are you receiving the most? The least?
    • Is it possible to get all the support you need from one person?
    • Which kinds of support are absolutely necessary for you to proceed and which are merely desirable?

9. Next, add your name to both lists. On the Supportive list, describe the ways in which you support your own fitness progress. On the Non-Supportive list, take stock of the ways you do not. Are you capable of doing for yourself what others cannot do?
    • Can you motivate yourself even when no one else can or will?
    • Overall, what support are you most lacking?
    • Do you need to make fitness more of a priority?
    • Do you need to stop letting others stop you?

10. Explore in your notebook any fears you have about how your new fitness journey may impact your relationships with family, friends, and cowork-ers. Include what you think their reactions might be (or already have been) to the changes in your behaviors, appearance, and attitudes.
    If you use food for emotional reasons, list which foods and situations set you up to overeat.

    _____

    _____

    _____

Check-In

1. How many days did you move for at least twenty minutes? Have you tried any of your favorite activities? Has it become easier or more enjoyable?

2. How many of the exercises at the end of the chapter have you been able to do? Which have been the most revealing? Which one did you avoid? Why? Do it anyway because it may be the one you would benefit from the most.

3. Have you wavered on the commitment you made to yourself in the beginning of the book or have you remained steady? Why or why not?

SECTION TWO

BRICKS & MORTAR

chapter four

Aerobic Program

So far, you've looked at past and present feelings about your body, exercise, diet, and at how others might have influenced you. You have the desire to move beyond past experiences and will soon see that you have the power. You've also moved your body twenty minutes or more each day with either familiar or new exercises. You've identified those activities you enjoy and why you enjoy them and now you have an opportunity to incorporate them into a structured, but not too structured, workout program.

The best workout program is flexible, realistic, backed by science, and authenticated by personal experience. Most importantly, it's one you like and one unique to you. The First Steps to Fitness program is designed to be that program. The next three chapters provide suggestions and guidelines on aerobic, weight, and diet training.

Before beginning the program, however, you may want to consult your doctor if you have any health concerns or are new to exercise.

Here are some important aerobic training facts:

1. Those who participate in regular cardiovascular activity at least three times per week live longer than those who do not.
2. To lose one pound, you have to burn or cut back 3,500 calories. The number of calories that cardiovascular and resistance training burns depends on your age, weight, sex, body fat percentage, and the intensity and duration of your workout.
3. Cardiovascular workouts strengthen your heart, which is a muscle that loses power, endurance, and strength if not exercised regularly.
4. Cardiovascular activity relieves stress, decreases depression, and increases well-being.

First Steps to Fitness Program

Schedule: Three days per week of cardiovascular movement

Time: 25–45 minutes

Intensity Level: For the aerobic workout to be most effective, exercise at the appropriate intensity level. A measure of intensity is target heart rate (THR), the rate at which you most efficiently burn body fat. Below is an example of a heart rate chart filled out by a forty-three-year-old.

TARGET HEART RATE CHART		
	220	This number is the maximum heart rate of a child at birth
Minus	43	Your age
Equals	177	Your maximum heart rate
Times	.70	Appropriate intensity level
Equals	124	Your target heart rate

She would do the main part of the workout at 124 beats per minute.

To calculate your target heart rate, plug your information into the boxes of the chart below:

TARGET HEART RATE CHART		
	220	This number is the maximum heart rate of a child at birth
Minus		Your age
Equals		Your maximum heart rate
Times	.70	Appropriate intensity level
Equals		Your target heart rate

No matter what aerobic activity you choose, begin with a five-minute warm-up. Then increase the intensity until you have achieved your THR and maintain it for the duration of your workout. Follow with a five-minute cool down.

Many cardio machines indicate your number of beats per minute. Another alternative is to use a heart rate monitor that straps around your chest. They are available at most gyms and sporting goods stores. If not on display at your gym, ask at the front desk.

Also, you can simply take your pulse halfway through your workout by finding your pulse on your wrist or neck and counting the beats for ten seconds. Then multiply this number by six and you will have your heart rate.

What if you are below your THR? Increase intensity through increased speed, resistance, or both until reaching your THR. You should be sweating, unable to easily carry on a conversation, and feel winded but not light-headed.

If you are one or two beats above your THR, don't worry. But if you are several beats above, then decrease your intensity until you reach your THR and maintain that level.

Below is a sample chart to use to plan and track your aerobic workouts (all blank charts can be found in the Appendix):

FIRST STEPS TO FITNESS AEROBIC PROGRAM

Before working out, how do I feel emotionally? Physically?

I'm tired but dedicated to losing weight.

Planned Program

Date:	Activity:	Time:
2/15	*bicycling*	
Warm Up:		5 minutes
Main Section:		15–35 min.
Cool Down:		5 minutes
Total Time:		25–45 min.

FIRST STEPS TO FITNESS AEROBIC PROGRAM

Completed Program

Date:	Activity:	Time:
2/15	bicycling	
Warm Up:		5 minutes
Main Section:		15 minutes
Cool Down:		5 minutes
Total Time:		25 min.

After working out, how do I feel emotionally? Physically?

Refreshed. I feel great!

Progress, not Perfection

Let's say you had your workout plan written, got started, and halfway through the workout realized it was too hard or too easy. No program is written in stone. As you go, you may have to increase or decrease the intensity. The important thing is to keep going. Track what you've done so you'll know what to do next time and so you can see where you've improved.

Selecting Forms of Aerobic Fitness

Do the aerobic activity of your choice. Clients who became fit faster performed aerobic activities they enjoyed and challenged themselves with progressively more difficult workouts than those who didn't. They looked forward to working out.

One client, Karen, enjoyed outdoor activities. She changed her routine seasonally. Every summer, she biked and ran outside. Every winter, she skied, ice skated, and used indoor cardio machines. She trained with weights year-round because she enjoyed them and found that it made her stronger for all the other activities she loved.

Sharon enjoyed hiking, so she created a hiking club. With a book detailing hundreds of hikes within fifty miles of where she lived, she and the club members would go on a different hike every week. Hiking past waterfalls, forests, mountains, and lakes, Sharon had a good time, lost weight and inches, felt better about herself, and developed friendships.

Diana used her competitive nature to her advantage. Every other month, her gym offered a different fitness competition, such as completing a certain number of miles on a cardio machine within a specified time. She entered every competition and won something each time. Her workouts never became stale, and her motivation stayed high.

Nicky ran three miles every day even though she didn't always enjoy it. She continued running because of the sense of accomplishment and the results—thinner thighs, flatter stomach, smaller clothes size. To remain motivated, she focused on what she liked about running rather than what she didn't.

In the first three chapters, you listed the physical activities you once enjoyed. Review these lists and then compile another one here of all the physical activities that you would like to do again or those you would like to try for the first time:

_____

_____

_____

Choose one or more to do in the next week.

Challenging Yourself

If you've been working out on the same machines or have attended the same aerobic classes for several months or even years, your body has become overaccustomed to the exercise and may have reached a plateau. Your workout may be easy. It may be fun. But it may not be challenging enough anymore to bring you the results you seek.

You may think, "It's hard enough to make working out a habit, but now you want me to keep changing my routine?" I know we are creatures of habit. Do the same cardio activity every day if you'd like, but if you get bored or for some other reason want to change, branch out. Try something on your list you haven't tried yet. Choose one day each week to do something different. If you've done step aerobics, try a cycling, yoga, kickboxing, or hip-hop class. Run a different route. Use a new machine. Just be careful to choose activities that are safe on your joints. Build up to more difficult activities. Roller blade on a flat surface a few times before attempting hills.

Try new things. Go at your own pace. Do what you enjoy.

Check-In

Do you have any reservations about the First Steps to Fitness Aerobics Program? If so, what is it? Is it something that you can change or overcome?

What, if anything, do you need to begin incorporating this part of the program into your life? For example, do you need to buy comfortable workout clothes or an exercise video?

chapter five

Weight-Training Program

In addition to aerobics, the First Steps to Fitness program includes an effective and efficient weight-training plan. Like most of my clients, you probably can't spend three or four hours a day in the gym pumping iron, even if you want to. Most likely, you aren't planning on becoming an international bodybuilding champion. If you are like my clients, you want to do what is necessary to firm, tone, add strength, and in general be healthier without spending too much time doing it. My clients found that the First Steps to Fitness weight-training program was realistic since it took only an hour twice per week and effective since they began to achieve the results they wanted in just a few weeks.

Resistance

Resistance training prepares your body for increasing challenges. You push yourself beyond what is comfortable so you can become stronger and more toned. Here are facts and experiences that I want to share with you.

1. To accomplish more in less time, exercise at a higher intensity level rather than for a longer duration.

    Many women's fitness magazines show pictures of eighteen-year-old girls lifting three-pound weights as if these light weights had toned their arms. This is false. Lifting a kitchen appliance or a small child is more work than that. To tone your arms, to get any of your muscles to respond to a workout, they must be challenged with a weight beyond what they normally lift.

2. A resistance training program must be progressively more challenging to see the changes that you want. The weight you lifted last week will be too easy for you next week.

    When I lifted light weights and performed fifteen or more repetitions of each exercise, my body didn't change. However, when I lifted heavier weights, increasing the weight by five or ten pounds every other session, a lot happened. In fact, I lost four sizes in four months.

3. Fat occupies much more space than muscle. According to Miriam Nelson, fitness director at Tufts University, a pound of fat is 30 percent larger than a pound of muscle. Many women fear "bulking up" from lifting weights, yet without taking muscle-building supplements or steroids, women won't develop big muscles because they don't have enough testosterone. Gaining muscle actually causes you to shrink.

   Occasionally I have had to stop lifting weights for several months and each time, my hips began to spread and my waist thickened even though I continued to watch my diet and do cardiovascular exercise. My weight went down, but my clothing size went up. I had lost muscle and gained fat. When I began to lift again, my body shrank back to my smaller size.

4. Muscle burns four times more calories than fat. Every pound of muscle burns an additional thirty to fifty more calories per day than fat. With increased muscles, you burn more calories during all activities, even sleeping, making it easier to lose or maintain your weight. According to Nelson, lifting weights may add two pounds of muscle every five to six weeks. This muscle would burn an additional sixty to one hundred calories per day. After twelve weeks, and another two pounds of muscle, you would burn an additional 120–200 calories per day.

   As you age (mid to late thirties and beyond), you lose about a half a pound of muscle each year. This leads to weight gain, fatigue, and loss of strength. However, you can avoid muscle loss with regular weight training.

5. Studies have shown that female aerobics instructors have more body fat than female bodybuilders. This is because too much cardiovascular exercise—more than five days per week for thirty minutes or more—can lead to muscle loss. When your body is forced to do a lot of pounding, such as with running or aerobics, it sheds heavy tissue (muscles) to make the body lighter. You begin to lose muscle rather than fat.

6. You also lose muscle when you excessively restrict your diet. When your calories are too low, your body doesn't have enough fuel to maintain

muscle tissue. Unfed muscles die. Remember that as you lose muscle, you lose calorie-burning capability, making weight control increasingly difficult. Reduce calories moderately (as you will with the First Steps to Fitness program), and incorporate resistance training into your routine. You will be able to lose fat and maintain muscle.

Special Populations

The fitness and health industry refers to individuals with special medical needs and concerns as special populations. People within these groups may still be able to lift weights and improve their health and well-being through weight training, but they need to modify their fitness routines to avoid injury and other medical problems.

The following is a list of conditions that classify individuals as part of a special population. If you have or suspect you might have any of these conditions, seek a physician's advice before beginning a weight-training program:

- High blood pressure
- Heart disease
- Cancer
- Pregnancy
- Extremely overweight or obese
- Diabetes
- Arthritis
- AIDS
- Over the age of fifty
- Under the age of eighteen
- Osteoporosis
- Asthma
- Injured or inflamed joints
- Any condition that requires medical attention

The First Steps to Fitness program is designed for those who are not part of a special population. If you have any of the above conditions or any other concerns about your state of health, talk to a physician. He or she can help you determine if you are ready to begin this program or if you need to modify it based on your circumstances.

First Steps to Fitness Weight-Training Program

Sets and Reps

How do you define sets and reps? A repetition (rep) is an individual completed movement, such as one biceps curl or one push-up. A set is a group of reps completed without rest. Ten push-ups in a row would be one set.

Breathing

When you are lifting the weight, breathe out. When lowering the weight, breathe in. Do not hold your breath because you could become light-headed, dizzy, or even faint, since breathing supplies your muscles with needed oxygen.

- Rest one minute between sets to allow muscles to re-energize.
- To prevent injury and to maintain control, lift to the count of four and lower in two.
- You may find padded lifting gloves, a water bottle, a sports watch, and a towel helpful.

Muscle groups targeted in each workout and examples of exercises (more information can be found in the Appendix):

Upper body

Muscles	Exercises
Chest	chest fly, dumbbell press
Back	bent-over rows, lat pull-downs, seated rows
Shoulder	lateral raises, overhead presses
Triceps (the back side of the upper arm, above the elbow joint and below the shoulder)	dips, French press, kickbacks, overhead extensions
Biceps (the front side of the upper arm, above the elbow joint and below the shoulder)	curls, preacher curls, concentration curls
Abdominal	various crunches with and without weight

Lower Body

Muscles	Exercises
Gluteus (the behind)	Squats, lunges
Quadriceps (the front side of the upper leg, above the knee joint and below the hip)	Extensions, squats
Inner Thigh	Inner thigh machines, leg lifts
Outer Thigh	Outer thigh machines, leg lifts
Hamstrings (the back side of the upper leg, above the knee joint and below the hip)	Hamstring curls
Calves	standing raises
Abdominal	various crunches with and without weights

Difficulty Level

Regardless of whether you are a beginner or a veteran at weight training, you will receive the best results if you are only able to lift the weight the prescribed number of reps for each set; if you can do more reps, the weight is too light. To determine the appropriate amount of weight you should lift for the greatest results, complete the Twelve-Rep Max Test for each exercise you choose to do. Every four weeks, when you switch to a new group of exercises, you will need to repeat this test. (If you are part of a special population, consult a physician before attempting the Twelve-Rep Max Test.)

Twelve-Rep Max Test

1. First, choose the exercises you want to do for the next four weeks and write them down on your workout sheets. For example, for your chest muscles you might select chest fly, for your back you might choose pull-downs, and for the front of the arm you might do biceps curls. See the Appendix for exercise descriptions and proper lifting instructions.

2. Then, start with the first exercise on your list. Warm up with a set of fifteen repetitions with light to moderate weight to lubricate muscles and joints.

3. Then, increase the weight by five to ten pounds. Lift, counting the number of repetitions you can do without resting between reps. You are finding out the maximum amount of weight you can lift only twelve times.

4. Rest thirty to sixty seconds and then increase the weight another five to ten pounds. Again, lift, counting the number of repetitions. When you reach a weight you can only lift twelve times, try another five to ten pounds more and see if you can also lift that weight twelve times. If not, then the previous amount was your Twelve-Rep Max. If you can lift the next weight twelve times, add another five to ten pounds and try again. For example, let's say you do a biceps curl with ten pounds for twelve reps, then you increase to fifteen pounds and do twelve reps again. You try twenty pounds and can only do eight reps. Now you know that your Twelve-Rep Max for that exercise is fifteen pounds. Stop the test if at any point along the way you feel joint pain or strain. If this happens, do not continue with the test. Instead, write down the amount of weight you were able to lift without any joint pain or strain as your starting weight.

5. Write down your Twelve-Rep Max amount, or other amount if you had joint pain, on your Week One workout sheets. Put the number on the Planned Program side, under the weight column. Every week thereafter, simply add five to ten pounds to your starting Twelve-Rep Max weight. (Add five pounds for small muscles like the biceps and triceps, ten pounds for larger muscles such as the hamstrings and gluteus.)

6. Repeat the above steps for each exercise you choose to do for the next four weeks.

The First Steps to Fitness Weight-Training Program consists of four-week segments. Two days per week are for weight training: one is for upper body, and one is for lower body. Each week is progressively more challenging, with fewer reps but increased sets and weight. At the end of the four weeks, you start over with week one, but with different exercises for each muscle group.

The schedule is as follows:

Week	Weight	Sets (groups of repetitions completed in a row without rest)	Reps (the number of completed repetitions of an exercise in a set)
One	Twelve-Rep Max	1–2	10–12
Two	Add 5–10 pounds to Twelve-Rep Max	2–3	8–10
Three	Add another 5–10 pounds	3–4	6–8
Four	Add another 5–10 pounds	4–5	4–6

The following sample charts include week one, lower body; and week two, upper body.

If you are currently doing no weight training or none consistently, then do the Week One routine for the entire first month instead of progressing through weeks Two, Three, and Four. This means you will do an upper body and a lower body workout once per week with two sets and ten to twelve reps of each exercise for your first month. This will prepare your muscles and joints to lift the heavier weights in the following weeks and reduce the risk of strain and injury.

After your first month, progress through the week Two, Three, and Four workouts.

FIRST STEPS TO FITNESS RESISTANCE PROGRAM
Week One Lower Body

Before I start, how do I feel physically? Emotionally?

I feel tired and stressed. I lack motivation.

Planned Program

Date:	8/15	Warm up:	5 minutes	
	Formula for Amount of Weight	Weight	Reps	Seconds Between Sets
Glute Exercise *Squats*	12-Rep Max Weight	50	10-12	60
	Same	50	10-12	0
Quadricep Exercise *Leg Extensions*	12-Rep Max Weight	40	10-12	60
	Same	40	10-12	0
Hamstring Exercise *Hamstring Curls*	12-Rep Max Weight	40	10-12	60
	Same	40	10-12	0
Inner Thigh Exercise *Inner Machine*	12-Rep Max Weight	70	10-12	60
	Same	70	10-12	0
Outer Thigh Exercise *Outer Machine*	12-Rep Max Weight	70	10-12	60
	Same	70	10-12	0
Calf Exercise *Standing Raises*	12-Rep Max Weight	30	10-12	60
	Same	30	10-12	0
Abdominal Exercise *Double Crunch*	12-Rep Max Weight	20	10-12	60
	Same	20	10-12	0
Lower Back Exercise *Extension*	12-Rep Max Weight	20	10-12	60
	Same	20	10-12	0

Stretches (Put a check when complete):	
Glute	√
Quadricep	√
Hamstring	√
Inner & Outer Thigh	√
Calf	√
Abdominal & Lower Back	√
Total Workout Time:	28 minutes

Completed Program			
Date:	8/15		
Warm up:	5 minutes		
	Weight	Reps	Seconds Between Sets
Glute Exercise	50	12	60
Squats	50	10	0
Quadricep Exercise	40	12	60
Leg Extensions	40	12	0
Hamstring Exercise	40	11	60
Hamstring Curls	40	10	0
Inner Thigh Exercise	70	12	60
Inner Machine	70	12	0
Outer Thigh Exercise	70	12	60
Outer Machine	70	12	0
Calf Exercise	30	12	60
Standing Raises	30	12	0
Abdominal Exercise	20	12	60
Double Crunch	20	10	0
Lower Back Exercise	20	12	60
Extension	20	11	0

Stretches (Put a check when complete):	
Glute	✓
Quadricep	✓
Hamstring	✓
Inner & Outer Thigh	✓
Calf	✓
Abdominal & Lower Back	✓
Total Workout Time:	29 min.

After working out, how do I feel emotionally? Physically?
I feel refreshed and rejuvenated.

FIRST STEPS TO FITNESS RESISTANCE PROGRAM
Week Two Upper Body

Before I start, how do I feel physically? Emotionally?

I feel okay. I'm looking forward to working out.

Planned Program

Date:	8/22	Warm up:	5 minutes		

	Formula for Amount of Weight	Weight	Reps	Seconds Between Sets
Chest Exercise	12-Rep Max Weight plus 5-10 lb.	40	8-10	60
	Same	40	8-10	60
Bench Press	Same	40	8-10	0
Back Exercise	12-Rep Max Weight plus 5-10 lb.	40	8-10	60
	Same	40	8-10	60
Back Row	Same	40	8-10	0
Shoulder Exercise	12-Rep Max Weight plus 5-10 lb.	30	8-10	60
	Same	30	8-10	60
Lateral Raise	Same	30	8-10	0
Tricep Exercise	12-Rep Max Weight plus 5-10 lb.	30	8-10	60
	Same	30	8-10	60
Pushdowns	Same	30	8-10	0
Bicep Exercise	12-Rep Max Weight plus 5-10 lb.	20	8-10	60
	Same	20	8-10	60
Curls	Same	20	8-10	0
Abdominal Exercise	12-Rep Max Weight plus 5-10 lb.	20	8-10	60
	Same	20	8-10	60
Basic Crunch	Same	20	8-10	0

Stretches (Put a check when complete):

Chest	√
Back	√
Shoulder	√
Tricep	√
Bicep	√
Abdominal	√
Total Workout Time:	36 minutes

Completed Program			
Date:			
Warm up:			
	Weight	Reps	Seconds Between Sets
Chest Exercise	40	8	60
	40	9	60
Bench Press	40	8	0
Back Exercise	40	10	60
	40	10	60
Back Row	40	9	0
Shoulder Exercise	30	8	60
	30	8	60
Lateral Raise	30	8	0
Tricep Exercise	30	9	60
Cable Press	30	9	60
Down	30	8	0
Bicep Exercise	20	10	60
	20	10	60
Bicep Curl	20	8	0
Abdominal Exercise	20	10	60
	20	10	60
Basic Crunch	20	10	0

Stretches (Put a check when complete):	
Chest	√
Back	√
Shoulder	√
Tricep	√
Bicep	√
Abdominal	√
Total Workout Time:	36 min.

After working out, how do I feel emotionally? Physically?

I feel refreshed and rejuvenated.

Progress, not Perfection

Sometimes you may be unable to perform all of the repetitions or lift all of the weight you've planned. It's the effort that is important. On your workout sheets, track not only what you planned to do, but also what you accomplished. This way, you can see your progress and where you may need to increase or decrease resistance.

Stretching

Each weight-training workout includes a five-minute section at the end for stretching. These stretches, shown along with the exercises in the Appendix, should be held for several seconds without bouncing. Relax into these stretches and breathe deeply. The goal is to end your workout session with your muscles lengthened and refreshed, not bound tighter than before you started.

Many people get injured (both during exercise and regular daily activities) because they do not stretch regularly. The most common muscles that are too tight and that are involved in most injuries are the hamstrings (back of the leg tightens up from sitting with knees bent all day), chest (shoulders round forward from sitting at a desk working on computers, talking on the phone, writing), lower back, and calves. A proper stretching routine can help prevent injuries.

Stretching regularly is even more important when you begin exercising because exercise causes muscles to tighten. If the muscles are not stretched, eventually the tightness leads to strain. Also, muscles have more ability to contract (meaning they are stronger) if they are flexible. Trying to get a tight muscle to contract is like trying to squeeze an orange that has already been squeezed dry. If you continue squeezing, it may fall apart. Inflexible muscles will weaken under stress. Joints attempt to compensate for the weakness, leading to injury.

Since incorporating stretching into the end of your routine is especially important, a stretching segment is included on all the workout sheets.

Emotional & Physical Inventory

The workout sheets include space for you to record your emotional and physical state both before and after exercising. By filling in this information, you'll see that working out makes you feel better.

Measurements

Since you will be doing resistance training, most of the time you will lose inches before losing pounds. Therefore, it is important to use measurements versus the scale to track your progress. At first, most clients dreaded measuring themselves, but after seeing results when they re-measured four weeks later, this became their favorite part. You measure to assess where you're starting from so later you can see how far you've come.

If you are overweight by more than seventy pounds, doing measurements may be counterproductive emotionally and mentally. You may choose instead to use the way your clothes feel as a guidepost until you lose some weight. Then, begin using measurements.

When and how do you measure?

When: every four weeks, approximately the same day and time. Measuring in the morning before eating is ideal because you're slightly dehydrated and not bloated from food, and you can get a more accurate measure of your true size. Also, if you measure about a week or two after your menstrual cycle, the measurements will be smaller due to less water retention.

How: Measure with a soft measuring tape. Pull the tape so that it is snug but not so tight that it changes the shape of the body. Don't be surprised if you find one side of your body bigger than the other. This is normal. Weight lifting often makes the two sides even.

- For the chest, bring the tape around your back and over the fullest part of your chest. Wear the same bra or no bra each time, as this will affect the measurements.

- For arms, wrap the tape around the widest part of your upper arm, usually a couple of inches below the armpit. Doing this measurement on yourself can be difficult. You may need to have someone else do this one for you. Or wrap a string around this part of your arm and without losing your place, lay the string out on the measuring tape to see how long it is.

- For abdominals, measure around your midsection, directly over your belly button.

- For hips/buttocks, stand with your feet together. Wrap the tape around the widest part of your buttocks. Stand in front of a mirror to see where you are measuring.

- For legs, stand with legs apart. Wrap the tape around the widest part of your legs, usually about an inch or two below the groin. Make sure you stand up as straight as you can before reading the measurement.

- For calves, wrap the tape around the widest part of your calf.

If you want to know how much body fat you have, have your body fat tested by a personal trainer or other health professional. Don't worry about what percentage the test indicates you have. It is not 100 percent accurate. Instead, focus on the difference between your first measurement and one done two to three months from now. For accurate comparison, the same person should perform the body fat test using the same technique.

The following is a sample chart filled in with the dates, times and measurements:

MEASUREMENT CHART

Date/Time:	Mon. 2/5 7am	Mon. 3/5 7am	+/−		+/−		+/−		+/−		+/−
Measurement			+/−		+/−		+/−		+/−		+/−	
Chest	38"	37"	−1									
Left Arm	12"	11"	−1									
Right Arm	12"	12"	0									
Abs (Belly Button)	36"	34"	−2									
Hip/Buttocks	40"	38"	−2									
Left Leg	25"	24"	−1									
Right Leg	25"	25"	0									
Left Calf	14"	13"	−1									
Right Calf	14"	13"	−1									
Total (+/-)			−9									

Check-In

It doesn't matter *where* you start. It only matters *that* you start.

1. Do you have any reservations about the First Steps to Fitness Weight Training program? If so, what are they? Are they things that you can change or overcome?

2. How do you feel about the results of your initial measurements or body fat test? Remember, we do this so we know where we started, not to make us feel bad. Be careful not to be too hard on yourself. Stay focused on the actions you plan to do to improve these measurements.

3. What, if anything, do you need to begin incorporating this part of the program into your life? For example, do you need to spend time reviewing the proper lifting techniques for each exercise and practicing the movements without weight before trying them with weight? Do you need to join a gym or buy some weight equipment to use at home?

chapter six

Eating Program

Just as I didn't tell you what kind of aerobic exercise to do, I'm not going to tell you what you should or shouldn't eat. You probably already know what is and what is not healthy. All I will do is show you a common-sense approach to eating to lose weight without feeling restricted. You will feel better, look better, and live healthier.

First Steps to Fitness Eating Program

The First Steps to Fitness program includes five main elements:

1. Total daily calories dependent upon your weight and goals
2. Daily calories divided into four or five small meals throughout the day
3. Filling foods (foods that keep blood sugar levels balanced, have high fiber, and combine carbohydrates, protein, and fat)
4. Eat moderately without feeling hungry
5. At least eight eight-ounce glasses of water per day

Let's start with the first element. Your total daily calorie intake depends upon how much you weigh and what you want to accomplish. Here is a simple and accurate calorie calculation: multiply your current weight by ten, twelve, or fifteen if you want to lose, maintain, or gain weight, respectively. This gives you the total daily calories you need. Next, divide your daily calories into five small meals.

The following chart shows the calculations for someone weighing 150 pounds who wants to lose weight.

CALORIE CALCULATION CHART

Current Weight	150
Multiply by 10 to lose, 12 to maintain, or 15 to gain	x 10
Total Daily Calories	1,500
Calories Per Meal (Daily cal. divided by 4 or 5)	300

CALORIE CALCULATION CHART

Current Weight	
Multiply by 10 to lose, 12 to maintain, or 15 to gain	
Total Daily Calories	
Calories Per Meal (Daily cal. divided by 4 or 5)	

As you lose weight, recalculate your calories. Let's say you went from 200 pounds to 180. Multiply your new weight by 10. Instead of two thousand calories per day, you'll need 1,800 to continue to lose. Once you reach your desired weight, multiply it by twelve to get the number of calories to maintain this weight.

Why does this program suggest so many meals? When eating two or three meals per day, you try to eat enough to provide energy for the whole day. But your body doesn't work like that. After a large meal, your digestion works over-time, which slows your metabolism. Whatever calories you consumed in excess of what you'll burn over the next three hours will be stored as fat. On the other hand, when you give your body just what it needs for the next three hours, it hums along like a sports car. Your metabolism is in high gear, and you feel energized and satisfied because you're using food to fuel activity.

Experiment by eating several small meals throughout the day for a few days and then switch to eating three big meals every day for a few days. Notice the difference in your energy level, digestion, and hunger level. Having five meals prevents you from overeating because you aren't allowing yourself to get too hungry.

Many people have complained that they couldn't lose weight even though they didn't eat very much. But they were only eating two or three times per day. Their metabolisms had slowed to ensure survival on infrequent meals. When they began to eat five small meals per day, every three hours, their metabolism sped up, they lost weight, they stored less body fat, and they felt satiated and healthier.

You may wonder how you will find time to prepare all of these meals. Most of the sample meals at the end of the chapter are simple to prepare. On days when you don't have much time, here are a few suggestions:

- While preparing lunch, for example, make an extra portion to use as another meal.
- Protein/energy shakes or bars (along with fruit and/or vegetables if desired) are easy, fast meals. Just beware of the sugar content of these items. Sometimes they have twenty-five grams or more per serving, which is enough to increase blood sugar levels and lead to fat storage and overeating.
- Have food in your car, at work, or in your purse that doesn't need to be refrigerated, such as canned tuna, fruit, soy nuts, protein bars, and beef or turkey jerky.
- Or carry a cooler stocked with foods such as sandwiches, yogurt, cheese, and more.

What if you hate counting calories? Rather than having to count calories all day, simply count by meal and keep in mind the number of meals you consume. This chapter provides examples of three-hundred-calorie meals to use or modify. In time, you'll automatically know which foods and in what amounts equal the calories you need. Also, you can splurge once per week and eat whatever you want.

Some clients hated counting calories, so they tried diet programs involving point systems or prepackaged meals in which the calorie calculations have already been done for them. By giving someone else responsibility for figuring out calories and amounts of foods, they didn't learn how to do it themselves. They generally did well as long as they ate the appropriate number of points or prepackaged foods, but as soon as they stopped, they gained the weight back. Sooner or later, they had to prepare their own food, count their own calories, and pay attention. There are two truths about weight loss: one, if you want to lose weight, you have to have a calorie deficit. There is no other way. Two, if you want to lose weight *for good*, you have to take personal responsibility for the necessary lifestyle changes.

Following is a sample First Steps to Fitness Eating Program sheet. You'll notice both the Planned Program and Completed Program sides are filled out. You may simply fill out the Completed side as you go rather than plan the day in advance, if you choose.

DAILY EATING PLAN

Planned Program

Date:	2/15			

MEAL ONE

Time	Food & Amounts	Calories	Fiber	Water
7 A.M.	Oatmeal, 1/3 c.	110	3	
Breakfast	Blueberries, 1 c.	82	4	
	Skim Milk, 1 c.	90	0	
	Total:	282	7	2 cups

MEAL TWO

Time	Food & Amounts	Calories	Fiber	Water
10 A.M.	Protein Bar, 1/2	150	0	
Snack	Carrots, 1 c.	48	4	
	Apricots, 1 c.	120	2	
	Total:	318	6	2 cups

MEAL THREE

Time	Food & Amounts	Calories	Fiber	Water
1 P.M.	Lunch Meat	100	0	
Lunch	Peas, 1/2 c.	60	4	
	Bread, 2 slices	100	2	
	1 tbsp. lite mayo	40	0	
	Total:	300	6	2 cups

MEAL FOUR

Time	Food & Amounts	Calories	Fiber	Water
4 P.M.	Strawberries, 1 c.	46	3.5	
Snack	Yogurt, lite 1 c.	100	0	
	Peanuts, 1/8 c.	107	1.5	
	Total:	253	5	2 cups

MEAL FIVE

Time	Food & Amounts	Calories	Fiber	Water
7 P.M.	Salmon, 4 oz.	200	0	
Dinner	Whole grain roll	100	1	
	Total:	300	1	1 cup

PLANNED

Total Daily Meals	Total Daily Calories	Total Daily Fiber	Total Daily Water
5	1,453 calories	25 grams	9 8 oz. glasses

Completed Program				
Date:	2/15			
MEAL ONE				
Time	Food & Amounts	Calories	Fiber	Water
7 A.M.	Oatmeal, 1/3 c.	110	3	
	Blueberries, 1/2 c.	41	2	
Breakfast	Skim Milk, 1 c.	90	0	
	Total:	241	5	2 cups
MEAL TWO				
Time	Food & Amounts	Calories	Fiber	Water
10 A.M.	Protein Bar, 1/2	150	0	
	Carrots, 1 c.	48	4	
Snack	Apricots, 1/2 c.	60	1	
	Total:	258	5	2 cups
MEAL THREE				
Time	Food & Amounts	Calories	Fiber	Water
1 P.M.	Lunch Meat	100	0	
	Peas, 1/2 c.	60	4	
Lunch	Bread, 2 slices	100	2	
	1 tbsp. lite mayo	40	0	
	Total:	300	6	2 cups
MEAL FOUR				
Time	Food & Amounts	Calories	Fiber	Water
4 P.M.	Strawberries, 1 c.	46	3.5	
	Yogurt, lite 1 c.	100	0	
Snack	Peanuts, 1/8 c.	107	1.5	
	Total:	253	5	2 cups
MEAL FIVE				
Time	Food & Amounts	Calories	Fiber	Water
7 P.M.	Salmon, 4 oz.	200	0	
	Whole grain roll	100	1	
Dinner				
	Total:	300	1	1 cup
COMPLETED				

Total Daily Meals	Total Daily Calories	Total Daily Fiber	Total Daily Water
5	1,352 calories	22 grams	9 8 oz. glasses

The fourth element of the First Steps to Fitness Eating Program involves food choices and ways to cut calories and eat moderately without feeling hungry.

First, combining carbohydrates, protein, and a little fat at each meal will satisfy you longer than having a meal of all carbohydrates, protein, or fat. Also, choose carbohydrates wisely. Richard N. Podell, M.D., author of *The G-Index Diet*, researched the effect carbs have on blood sugar and weight loss. Certain carbs (called high-glycemic) cause a sharp rise in blood sugar levels after eating, which then leads to a crash in blood sugar that causes cravings for more food. Other carbs (called low-glycemic) cause only a slight increase in blood sugar and therefore do not lead to overeating.

Which foods are high-glycemic and which are low? Unfortunately and not coincidentally, most foods people tend to love and crave are high-glycemic: refined-flour breads, chips, crackers, sweets, baked white potatoes. However, if you choose to eat a high-glycemic food such as carrots or white bread, minimize the rise in your blood sugar by mixing the food with something low-glycemic, such as fat or protein.

The following foods are highest in glycemic value, meaning they will cause a sharp rise in blood sugar, which leads to increased body fat storage and food cravings (minimize these foods in your diet):

HIGH-GLYCEMIC FOODS
- Products made from refined flour, such as bread, cakes, muffins, biscuits, rolls
- Sugar in all forms (except fructose): granulated, honey, molasses, syrup
- Bananas and tropical fruits such as papaya, mango, pineapple
- Cereals
- White potatoes

The following foods are lowest in glycemic value. These foods will keep blood sugar balanced, which helps increase satiety, decrease overeating, and improve your ability to burn fat and lose weight (select these for your meals). Scan the chart and ask yourself if you have ever binged on any of these foods:

LOW-GLYCEMIC FOODS
- Meats
- Milk
- All whole grains, including whole oats (not quick-cooking), barley, buckwheat, couscous
- Vegetables (except carrots and baked potatoes)
- North American fruits, such as berries and apples
- Sweet potatoes

High-glycemic foods burn quickly and leave you feeling hungry soon after you have eaten. They also cause craving for more high-glycemic foods. Here's an experiment you can do to see for yourself how high-glycemic food affects your blood sugar levels and your hunger: eat something high-glycemic, such as a piece of bread with honey on it or a banana. Don't mix this food with low-glycemic or high-fat foods. Pay attention to how long it takes before you are hungry again.

In contrast, low-glycemic foods keep you feeling satisfied and less hungry and do not lead to cravings and overeating. Experiment to see how low-glycemic foods affect your blood sugar. Eat something low-glycemic, such as a piece of meat, egg whites, or a half-cup of whole grains (slow-cooking oats, whole barley, wheat berries). Don't mix your selection with high-glycemic foods. How long before you feel hungry? Compare this time frame to what happened when you ate the high-glycemic food.

Equally important in food selection is the amount of fiber. Fiber has few or no calories. It also fills you up because it keeps your digestion busy. The average person consumes only ten to twelve grams of fiber per day. Nutritionists recommend twenty to thirty grams per day. Work your way up slowly, adding a few grams of fiber each day until you reach approximately five grams or more per meal. This will help you avoid the intestinal stress fiber can cause.

Following is a list of high-fiber foods:

FOOD	AMOUNT	FIBER
Lentils	1/2 cup	5 grams
Black beans	1/2 cup	6 grams
Refried beans	1/2 cup	6 grams
Apples	one	3 grams
Pear	one	4 grams
Strawberries	1 cup	3 grams
Oats	1/3 cup dry	3 grams
Soybeans (roasted)	1/4 cup	4 grams
Sweet potato (baked)	one	3.4 grams
Lettuce	9 large leaves	3 grams
Peas	1/2 cup	4 grams
High-fiber breakfast cereal such as:		
Oatmeal	1 cup	8 grams
Kellogg's All Bran	1/2 cup	10 grams
Post Raisin Bran	1 cup	8 grams
Nuts	1/4 cup	3 grams
Flax Seeds	2 tbsp	3 grams

To help the fiber move through your digestive track, drink plenty of water. The First Steps to Fitness program calls for at least eight eight-ounce servings spread out evenly throughout the day. Drinking this amount or more every day also helps you lose inches by alleviating water retention and curbing appetite.

Many clients balked at the suggestion of drinking more water. "But I hate the taste," they'd say, or "I'll have to run to the bathroom all day if I drink that much," or "I'm not thirsty, so why should I drink it?" You may have these same objections. Let's take one at a time.

Our taste buds become so used to overly sweet beverages, it takes time to read-just to plain water. The better the water, the better the taste, so check into bottled spring water. Also, squeezing a lemon, lime, or orange into your water may make it more palatable.

Drinking a lot of water does require more trips to the bathroom. However, spreading the water out evenly throughout the day helps minimize mad dashes to the restroom. The benefits of drinking water outweigh this inconvenience.

If you wait until you're thirsty to drink water, you've waited too long because you already have a water deficit. The idea is to have a continuous water *surplus* to obtain the benefits, such as decreased water retention.

The following are more benefits of drinking plenty of water:
- Suppresses the appetite
- Helps the body metabolize stored fat
- Decreases fatigue and moodiness
- Increases muscular performance
- Regulates body temperature
- Improves blood circulation
- Helps eliminate toxins and waste from the body

Other liquids don't count as water. Caffeinated beverages cause dehydration. Liquids containing sugar or fruit juice have to be digested, and since digestion requires water, these drinks cause a greater water deficit.

Here are a few tips for tracking the amount of water that you drink in a day:
1. Use a water bottle and fill it throughout the day. (The larger the bottle, the fewer times you have to refill it and the easier it is to track.)
2. Around the neck of the bottle, wrap a number of rubber bands that corresponds with the number of times you plan to refill the bottle (if it is a sixteen-ounce bottle, you'd fill it four to six times). Each time you finish the bottle, remove one of the rubber bands.
3. Drink half of your daily amount by noon and the other half by 6 P.M. to avoid midnight trips to the bathroom.

How many cups of caffeinated coffee, soda, and tea do you drink daily? Caffeine is a double-edged sword: on one hand, it stimulates the central nervous system, increases the speed at which you burn calories, mobilizes free fatty acids, and improves muscle contractions. On the other hand, it dehydrates the body. Dehydration causes fatigue, decreased muscular performance, moodiness, and more. Also, often people confuse hunger for thirst and end up eating instead of drinking water.

Each of us has a different tolerance level for caffeine. Pay attention to how you feel an hour or two after ingesting caffeine. Are you thirsty? Hungry? Jittery? Tired? If you don't have caffeine, do you go through withdrawals and experience headaches or moodiness?

How do you cut back if you're drinking two pots of coffee per day or several sodas? When I decided to avoid caffeine, I was drinking four to six cups of regular coffee daily and one large soda. I started by drinking half regular and half decaf coffee, gradually increasing the decaf grounds. I cut out the soda when I realized how thirsty I felt after drinking it. Moderation is key. Now, if I have caffeine, I have only one cup of regular coffee in a day.

Caffeine is a drug. Just as with nicotine, alcohol, or other substances, ask yourself why you have it. Are you often tired? If yes, why? Is there anything you can do to feel less tired besides ingest caffeine?

Let's talk about another drug, alcohol. When my clients wrote down the amount of calories they consumed in a week, many of them left out alcoholic beverages. They didn't think of alcohol as having calories. Yet alcohol has almost as many calories per gram as fat! Alcohol has seven calories per gram, and fat has nine.

A twelve-ounce can of regular beer packs one hundred and fifty calories. Light beer has one hundred. Two tablespoons of hard liquor such as gin, rum, vodka, or whiskey has seventy calories.

So let's say you go out on Friday night and have a glass of wine with dinner (seventy calories) and one light beer (one hundred calories). Then on Saturday, you have two mixed drinks at a bar (two hundred and eighty calories). This would be an extra four hundred and ten calories. If you did this every weekend, you would gain a half of a pound a month from alcohol alone. How many calories do you consume from alcohol in a week or a month?

Sample 300-Calorie Meals

If you're not used to preparing small meals, don't worry. Below are lists of meals for breakfast, lunch, dinner, and snacks. They are all within the three-hundred-calorie range so you may need to add or subtract foods or increase or decrease serving sizes, depending on your calorie needs. The meals are primarily low-glycemic, high-fiber, and balanced between protein, carbohydrates, and fat. Vegetarian meals are marked by a *V*. The meals are interchangeable. You can have a breakfast meal for lunch, and so on. Simply prepare the provided meals, make substitutions, or create your own. If unfamiliar with the caloric content of foods, you can find books that provide these details or locate the information online.

Breakfast Meal Ideas

Foods	Serving Size	Calories	Fiber	Carbohydrate	Protein	Fat
Veggie omelet (V)						
Canned mushrooms	1/4 cup	12	1	X		
Tomatoes	1/4 cup	10	0.5	X		
Bread	2 slices	100	2	X		
Apple	1	80	3	X		
Egg whites	3/4 cup	105	0		X	
Meal Total:		**307**	**6.5**			
Bagel egg sandwich (V)						
Multigrain bagel	1	150	3	X		
Whole egg	1	86	0		X	X
Low-fat cheese	1 slice	45	0		X	X
Berries	1/2 cup	40	2	X		
Meal Total:		**321**	**5**			
Cereal & fruit (V)						
High-fiber cereal	1 cup	130	10	X		
Strawberries	1 cup	46	3.4	X		
Skim milk	1 1/2 cup	120	0	X	X	
Meal Total:		**296**	**13.4**			

Foods	Serving Size	Calories	Fiber	Carbohydrate	Protein	Fat
Scrambled eggs (V)						
Canned mushrooms	1/4 cup	12	1	X		
Canned black beans	1/4 cup	50	3	X	X	
Bread	1 slice	50	1	X		
Egg whites	3/4 cup	105	0		X	
Low-fat cheese	1 slice	45	0		X	X
Meal Total:		**262**	**5**			
Cottage cheese & fruit (V)						
Pineapple	1/2 cup	70	1	X		
Berries	1 cup	80	4	X		
Cottage cheese 1%	1 cup	164	0		X	X
Meal Total:		**314**	**5**			
PB&J (V)						
Bread	1 slice	50	1	X		
All-fruit jelly	1 tbsp	40	0	X		
Milk	3/4 cup	60	0	X	X	
Peanut butter	1 tbsp	100	1		X	X
Orange	1	65	3.4	X		
Meal Total:		**250**	**5.4**			
Salsa scramble (V)						
Salsa	2 tbsp	10	1	X		
Bread	1 slice	50	1	X		
Egg whites	1/2 cup	70	0		X	
Low-fat cheese	1 slice	45	0		X	X
Dried fruit	1/3 cup	110	5	X		
Meal Total:		**285**	**6**			

Foods	Serving Size	Calories	Fiber	Carbohydrate	Protein	Fat
Bagel & cream cheese (V)						
Multigrain bagel	1	150	3	X		
Cream cheese	2 tbsp	100	0		X	X
Jelly/preserves	1 tbsp	50	0	X		
Meal Total:		**300**	**3**			
Oatmeal & raisins (V)						
Oatmeal	1/2 cup	140	4	X		
Raisins	2 tbsp	65	1	X		
Milk	1 cup	80	0	X	X	
Meal Total:		**285**	**5**			
Pancakes (V)						
Pancakes	2 pcs	150	1	X		
Light syrup	2 tbsp	50	0	X		
Berries	1 1/4 cup	100	5	X		
Meal Total:		**300**	**6**			
Eggs & sausage						
Bread	1 slice	50	1	X		
Egg whites	1/2 cup	70	0		X	
Light sausage links	1 link	110	0		X	X
Apple	1	80	3.4	X		
Meal Total:		**310**	**4.4**			
Health shake & fruit (V)						
Berries	11/2 cup	120	6	X		
Protein shake mix	1 scoop	85	0		X	
Low-fat yogurt	1 cup	100	0	X	X	
Meal Total:		**305**	**6**			

Lunch Meal Ideas

Foods	Serving Size	Calories	Fiber	Carbohydrate	Protein	Fat
Tuna sandwich (V)						
Lettuce	3 large leaves	6	1	X		
Bread	2 slices	100	2	X		
Tuna	1 3-oz. can	100	0		X	
Light mayonnaise	1 tbsp	40	0		X	
Strawberries	1 cup	46	3.4			X
Meal Total:		**292**	**6.4**			
Turkey sandwich						
Cauliflower/broccoli, raw	1 cup	25	2.6	X		
Bread	2 slices	100	2	X		
Lean turkey lunch meat	4 slices	92	0		X	
Mustard	1/2 tbsp	10	0	X		
Milk	1 cup	80	0	X	X	
Meal Total:		**307**	**4.6**			
Ham & cheese						
Dark green lettuce	3 large leaves	6	1	X		
Bread	2 slices	100	2	X		
Baby raw carrots	5 medium	20	2	X		
Extra lean ham sliced thin	3 slices	111	0		X	
Mustard	1/2 tbsp	10	0	X		
Cheese	1 slice	45	0		X	X
Meal Total:		**292**	**5**			

Foods	Serving Size	Calories	Fiber	Carbohydrate	Protein	Fat
Boiled egg (V)						
Celery stalk, raw	3 large stalks	18	2	X		
Bread	2 slices	100	2	X		
Pear	1	98	4	X		
Boiled egg	1	86	0		X	X
Meal Total:		**302**	**8**			
Chicken sandwich						
Dark green lettuce	6 large leaves	12	2	X		
Carrots	1/2 cup sliced	20	2	X		
Whole grain bun	1	100	2	X		
Lean chicken breast, no skin	1	150	0		X	X
Meal Total:		**282**	**6**			
Meatless burger (V)						
Bread	2 slices	100	2	X		
Boca Burger (meatless)	1	90	4	X	X	
Light cheese	1 slice	45	0		X	X
Apple	1	80	3	X		
Meal Total:		**315**	**9**			
Turkey sausage						
Hot dog bun	1	100	1	X		
Peas	1/2 cup	60	4	X		
Lean turkey Italian sausage	1	140	0		X	X
Ketchup & mustard	1 tsp each	15	0	X		
Meal Total:		**315**	**5**			

Foods	Serving Size	Calories	Fiber	Carbohydrate	Protein	Fat
Stuffed potato						
Broccoli or 1 cup cauliflower, raw	25	2.6	X			
Potato with skin	1	220	4.8	X		
Light cheese	1 slice	45	0		X	X
Lean turkey lunch meat	1 slice	23	0		X	
Meal Total:		**313**	**7.4**			
Lentils & rice (V)						
Lentils	1 cup	172.5	11.7	X	X	
Rice (brown or white)	1/2 cup	104	0.5	X		
Meal Total:		**276.5**	**12.2**			
Hummus wrap (V)						
Hummus	2 ounces	170	2			
Bell peppers	1/2 pepper sliced	10	0.65	X		
Lettuce	1 large leaf	2	0.3			
Cucumber	1/2 cup sliced	7	0.4			
Flour tortilla	6 inch	100	1	X		
Meal Total:		**289**	**4.35**			
Bean soup & crackers (V)						
Bean soup	1 cup	130	3			
Crackers	5	70	0.5			
Apple	1	80	3			
Meal Total:		**280**	**6.5**			

Dinner Meal Ideas

Foods	Serving Size	Calories	Fiber	Carbohydrate	Protein	Fat
Grilled/broiled fish (V)						
Dark green lettuce	6 large leaves torn	12	2	X		
Green onion (scallions)	1/2 cup chopped	16	1.3	X		
Italian bread crumbs to coat	1 tbsp	27.5	0	X		
Salmon, swordfish or other	3 oz (palm size)	130	0		X	X
Olive oil to coat fish	1/2 tbsp	50	0			X
Low-fat dressing	1 tbsp	15	0	X		X
Garlic salt to shake on fish	1 tsp	0	0	X		
Peas	1/2 cup	60	4	X		
Meal Total:		**310.5**	**7.3**			
Turkey shish kabob						
Bell pepper	1 whole sliced	20	1.3	X		
Onion	1 whole cubed	20	1	X		
Zucchini	1/2 cup sliced	9	0.8	X		
Fresh mushrooms	1/2 cup	9	0.4	X		
Lean turkey breast no skin	3 oz (palm size)	160	0		X	X
Olive oil to drizzle on kabob	1/2 tbsp	50	0			X
Poultry seasoning	2 tsp	0	0	X		
Corn	1/4 cup	40	1	X		
Meal Total:		**308**	**4.5**			

Foods	Serving Size	Calories	Fiber	Carbohydrate	Protein	Fat
Chicken stir fry						
Carrots	1/2 cup sliced	20	2	X		
Bell peppers	1/2 pepper sliced	10	0.65	X		
Rice (brown or white)	1/4 cup	52	0.25	X		
Lean chicken breast no skin	1	150	0		X	X
Canola oil	1/2 tbsp	50	0			X
Soy sauce	1 tbsp	10	0	X		
Sugar snap peas	1/2 cup	20	2	X		
Meal Total:		**312**	**4.9**			
Turkey burrito						
Dark green lettuce	3 large leaves torn	6	1	X		
Flour tortilla	6 inch	100	1	X		
Nonfat refried beans	1/4 cup	55	3	X	X	
Lean ground turkey	3 oz (palm size)	112	0		X	X
Light cheese	1 slice	45	0		X	X
Meal Total:		**318**	**5**			
Black bean salad (V)						
Pasta	1 cup	197	2.4	X		
Black beans	1/2 cup	90	4	X	X	
Parmesan cheese	1 tbsp	20	0		X	X
Asparagus	2 spears sliced	7	0.6	X		
Meal Total:		**314**	**7**			

Foods	Serving Size	Calories	Fiber	Carbohydrate	Protein	Fat
Lean burgers						
Dark green lettuce	2 large leaves	4	1	X		
Onion	3 slices	10	0	X		
Whole grain bun	1	100	2	X		
Lean ground chicken	3 oz (palm size)	112.5	0		X	X
Canned green beans	1/2 cup	30	2	X		
Low-fat mayonnaise	1/2 tbsp	20	0			X
Mustard	1/2 tbsp	10	0	X		
Tomato	1/4 cup sliced	9.5	0.5	X		
Ketchup	1/2 tbsp	7.5	0	X		
Meal Total:		**303.5**	**5.5**			
Steak & potato						
Dark green lettuce	6 large leaves torn	12	2	X		
Raw carrots	1/4 cup sliced	10	1	X		
Potato with skin	1/4 potato	36.5	1	X		
Canned mushrooms	1/4 cup	6	0.5	X		
Lean beef tenderloin	3 oz (palm size)	247	0		X	X
Low-fat salad dressing	1/2 tbsp	7.5	0	X		
Low-fat sour cream	1/2 tbsp	10	0			X
Meal Total:		**329**	**4.5**			

Foods	Serving Size	Calories	Fiber	Carbohydrate	Protein	Fat
Tofu stir-fry (V)						
Raw carrots	1/2 cup sliced	20	2	X		
Bell pepper	1 sliced	20	1.3	X		
Celery	1 1/2 large stalks	9	1	X		
Rice (brown or white)	1/2 cup	108	0.5	X		
Firm tofu	1/5 of 1 lb block	90	0		X	X
Soy sauce	1 tbsp	10	0	X		
Olive or canola oil for cooking	1/2 tbsp	50	0			X
Meal Total:		**307**	**4.8**			
Ham Wrap						
Dark green lettuce	3 large leaves	6	1	X		
Tomato	1/2 cup sliced	19	0.5	X		
Flour tortilla	6 inch	100	1	X		
Extra lean ham sliced thin	3 slices	111	0		X	X
Light cheese	1 slice	45	0		X	X
Mustard	1/2 tbsp	10	0	X		
Celery	3 large stalks	18	2	X		
Meal Total:		**309**	**4.5**			

Foods	Serving Size	Calories	Fiber	Carbohydrate	Protein	Fat
Homemade pizza						
Pizza sauce	4 tbsp	30	1	X		
Green onion (scallions)	1/4 cup 8 chopped	0.65	X			
Canned mushrooms	1/4 cup sliced	12	1	X		
Lean turkey Italian sausage	1/2 medium	70	0		X	X
Light cheese	2 tbsp grated	50	0		X	X
Pizza crust	1 slice	100	0.5	X		
Lettuce	6 large leaves torn	12	2	X		
Low-fat salad dressing	1 tbsp	14	0	X		
Meal Total:		**296**	**5.15**			
Big chicken salad						
Dark green lettuce	8 large leaves torn	16	1.5	X		
Tomato	1/2 cup chopped	19	0.5	X		
Green onion (scallions)	1/2 cup 16 chopped	1.3	X			
Raw carrots	1/2 cup sliced	20	2	X		
Lean chicken breast, no skin	1	150	0		X	X
Croutons	2 tbsp	30	0	X		
Low-fat dressing	2 tbsp	30	0	X		
Sunflower seeds	1/2 tbsp	23	0.5			X
Meal Total:		**304**	**5.8**			

Foods	Serving Size	Calories	Fiber	Carbohydrate	Protein	Fat
Salad with tuna (V)						
Dark green lettuce	8 large leaves, torn	16	1.5	X		
Green onion (scallions)	1/2 cup chopped	16	1.3	X		
Berries	1 cup	80	4	X		
Croutons	2 tbsp	30	0	X		
Tuna	1–3 oz can	100	0		X	
Parmesan cheese	1 tbsp	20	0		X	X
Olive oil	1/2 tbsp	50	0			X
Meal Total:		**312**	**6.8**			
Veggie burgers (V)						
Dark green lettuce	2 large leaves	4	1	X		
Onion	3 slices	10	0	X		
Whole grain bun	1	100	2	X		
Veggie burger	1 patty	100	4		X	X
Canned green beans	1/2 cup	30	2	X		
Low-fat mayonnaise	1/2 tbsp	20	0			X
Mustard	1/2 tbsp	10	0	X		
Tomato	1/4 cup sliced	9.5	0.5	X		
Ketchup	1/2 tbsp	7.5	0	X		
Meal Total:		**291**	**9.5**			

Snack Meal Ideas

Foods	Serving Size	Calories	Fiber	Carbohydrate	Protein	Fat
Apple & peanut butter (V)						
Apple	1	60	3	X		
Light yogurt	1 cup	100	0	X	X	
Peanut butter	1 1/2 tbsp	150	1			X
Meal Total:		**310**	**4**			
Trail mix (V)						
Raisins	2 tbsp	65	1	X		
Whole oats	1/4 cup	70	2	X		
Any kind of nuts	1 tbsp	45	0.75		X	X
Soy nuts	1/4 cup	120	4	X	X	X
Meal Total:		**300**	**7.75**			
Cottage cheese & fruit (V)						
Cottage cheese 1%	1 cup	164	0		X	X
Pineapple	1/2 cup	70	1	X		
Berries	1 cup	80	4	X		
Meal Total:		**314**	**5**			
Celery & cream cheese (V)						
Banana	1	138	2	X		
Raw celery stalks	3 large stalks	18	2	X		
Light cream cheese	4 tbsp (1/4 cup)	140	0	X	X	X
Meal Total:		**296**	**4**			
Veggies & string cheese (V)						
Raw broccoli or cauliflower	1 cup	25	2.6	X		
Raw baby carrots	10 medium	40	4	X		
Low-fat string cheese	3 pcs	240	0		X	X
Asparagus	8 spears	28	2.6	X		
Meal Total:		**305**	**9.2**			

Foods	Serving Size	Calories	Fiber	Carbohydrate	Protein	Fat
Chips, cheese & salsa (V)						
Salsa	3 tbsp	15	1.5	X		
Low-fat tortilla chips	1 oz	130	1	X		
Low-fat string cheese	1 piece	80	0		X	X
Nonfat refried beans	1/4 cup	55	3		X	
Meal Total:		**280**	**5.5**			
Soy nuts & fruit (V)						
Apple	1	60	3	X		
Roasted soy nuts	1/2 cup	240	8	X	X	X
Meal Total:		**300**	**11**			
Cottage cheese, fruit, seeds (V)						
Apricots	1 cup	74	2	X		
Cottage cheese 1%	3/4 cup	123	0		X	X
Sunflower seeds	1 tbsp	46.5	0.5		X	X
Berries	1/2 cup	40	2	X		
Meal Total:		**283.5**	**4.5**			
Bagel & cream cheese (V)						
Raw broccoli or cauliflower	1 cup	25	2.6	X		
Raw cucumber	1 cup sliced	14	0.8	X		
Multigrain bagel	1	150	3	X		
Light cream cheese	3 tbsp	105	0		X	X
Meal Total:		**294**	**6.4**			
Protein—energy bar & fruit (V)						
Pear	1	98	4	X		
Celery	6 large stalks	36	4	X		
Protein—energy bar	1/2 bar	150	0		X	
Meal Total:		**284**	**8**			

Foods	Serving Size	Calories	Fiber	Carbohydrate	Protein	Fat
Protein drink with fruit (V)						
Cantaloupe	1/2 cup	29	0.6	X		
Protein shake mix	1 scoop	85	0		X	
Low-fat yogurt	3/4 cup	75	0		X	X
Flax seeds	2 tbsp	70	3			X
Berries	1/2 cup	40	2	X		
Meal Total:		**299**	**5.6**			
Protein bar & milk (V)						
Protein Bar	1/2 bar	150	0		X	
Milk	1 cup	80	0	X	X	
Berries	1 cup	80	4	X		
Meal Total:		**310**	**4**			

Splurge Days

So does all this mean you can't ever eat a piece of cake or have a glass of wine? No, because this program includes one day out of the week in which you can splurge—eat whatever you want without counting calories or meals. Friday, Saturday, or whatever day you expect to feel most tempted make the best Splurge Days. The day you splurge could be different each week, just be sure you plan for it so you have something to look forward to and so you keep it to one day. Having one higher-calorie day in the week helps you boost your metabolism, build muscle, and mentally commit to the low-calorie days. Enjoy yourself.

Progress, not Perfection

Adjusting to this eating program may take some time. One client was excited about having a Splurge Day each week but said having small meals would be challenging because she was used to large meals and was afraid she'd be hungry. She discovered it wasn't as difficult as she anticipated because she only had to wait three hours before eating again. And filling up with fiber and low-glycemic foods made it easy for her to stay full until the next meal.

Give yourself at least a week or two to become comfortable with this program. If after that time you still can't seem to fit in five meals a day, divide the number of calories you need into three or four meals. If you can't eat twenty-five grams of fiber per day or complete some other part of the plan, don't worry. Do what you can. This program is flexible so that you can fit it into your life and achieve the results you seek.

Check-In

1. Have you been following your First Steps to Fitness aerobic and weight training programs? How do you feel?

2. What is your biggest concern about the eating program? Is it something you can overcome? Are you willing to be patient with yourself as you make these changes?

chapter seven

Program Schedule

Now, you may be wondering how you will schedule your workout program. When will you do aerobic and weight training? In the morning, afternoon, or evening? Maybe you'll only work out on weekends. There is not a right or wrong time; only the time that works best for you.

In addition to the workout and meal sheets, there are also schedule sheets for weekly planning and tracking. You may have a fairly predictable weekly schedule, so you can plan the month and quarter in advance. Or you may have a less predictable schedule and may feel comfortable planning only one week at a time. Either approach works.

Following is a sample Schedule Sheet of an exerciser with a predictable, consistent schedule. (We will discuss the Rewards and Goals columns in the next chapter.)

		MON.	TUES.	WED.	THURS.	FRI.	SAT.	SUN.	Weekly Goals		Weekly Rewards	
WEEK												
WEEK 1	WORK-OUT TYPE	Weights Upper Body		Weights Lower Body	Cardio	Cardio	Cardio	Rest Day				
	MEAL PLAN	5 meals 1400 calories	5 meals 1400 calories	5 meals 1400 calories	5 meals 1400 calories	5 meals 1400 calories	Splurge Day	5 meals 1400 calories				
WEEK 2	WORK-OUT TYPE	Weights Upper Body		Weights Lower Body	Cardio	Cardio	Cardio	Rest Day				
	MEAL PLAN	5 meals 1400 calories	5 meals 1400 calories	5 meals 1400 calories	5 meals 1400 calories	5 meals 1400 calories	Splurge Day	5 meals 1400 calories				

SCHEDULE SHEET

SCHEDULE SHEET												
WEEK		MON.	TUES.	WED.	THURS.	FRI.	SAT.	SUN.	Weekly Goals		Weekly Rewards	
WEEK 3	WORK-OUT TYPE	Weights Upper Body		Weights Lower Body	Cardio	Cardio	Cardio	Rest Day				
	MEAL PLAN	5 meals 1400 calories	5 meals 1400 calories	5 meals 1400 calories	5 meals 1400 calories	5 meals 1400 calories	Splurge Day	5 meals 1400 calories				
WEEK 4	WORK-OUT TYPE	Weights Upper Body		Weights Lower Body	Cardio	Cardio	Cardio	Rest Day				
	MEAL PLAN	4–5 meals 1400 calories	4–5 meals 1400 calories	4–5 meals 1400 calories	4–5 meals 1400 calories	4–5 meals 1400 calories	Splurge Day	4–5 meals 1400 calories				

Monthly Goals:	Quarterly Goals:	Annual Goals:
Monthly Rewards:	Quarterly Rewards:	Annual Rewards:

The following is a sample workout Schedule Sheet of an exerciser with an unpredictable schedule. She doesn't exercise on the same days each week, so she plans one week at a time.

SCHEDULE SHEET										
WEEK		MON.	TUES.	WED.	THURS.	FRI.	SAT.	SUN.	Weekly Goals	Weekly Rewards
WEEK 1	WORK-OUT TYPE	Cardio	Cardio	Weights Lower Body	Weights Upper Body		Cardio			
	MEAL PLAN	5 meals 1200 calories	5 meals 1200 calories	5 meals 1200 calories	5 meals 1200 calories	5 meals 1200 calories	Splurge Day	5 meals 1200 calories		
WEEK 2	WORK-OUT TYPE	Weights Upper Body		Weights Lower Body	Cardio	Cardio		Cardio		
	MEAL PLAN	5 meals 1200 calories	5 meals 1200 calories	5 meals 1200 calories	5 meals 1200 calories	5 meals 1200 calories	5 meals 1200 calories	Splurge Day		

SCHEDULE SHEET

WEEK		MON.	TUES.	WED.	THURS.	FRI.	SAT.	SUN.	Weekly Goals	Weekly Rewards
WEEK 3	WORK-OUT TYPE									
	MEAL PLAN									
WEEK 4	WORK-OUT TYPE									
	MEAL PLAN									

Monthly Goals:	Quarterly Goals:	Annual Goals:
Monthly Rewards:	Quarterly Rewards:	Annual Rewards:

Check-In

1. How many days this week did you complete your workout and eating plans?

2. Have you tried any new physical activities or any from your "favorites" list?

Constructing & Maintaining Your Dream "House"

chapter eight

Goals and Rewards

You have created an excellent foundation on which to build. Now what kind of house will you build on that foundation? Where do you want to be in two months, six months, one year? In this chapter, you'll imagine what you want to look like, how you want to feel, think, and behave. The power of the imagination is great. Prisoners of war often talk about how, while imprisoned in deplorable conditions, they turned to their imaginations to cope. They would envision in great detail the house they wanted to build, or the boat, or the business. Amazingly, when they returned home, they were often able, brick by brick, to replicate what they had constructed in their minds. If you apply even a fraction of this effort to creating the body you want, just imagine what could happen.

Within the first four to six weeks, those who follow the First Steps to Fitness program on average lose 1 to 1.5 percent body fat and four and a half inches overall, primarily from their hips, thighs, and abdomen. And this is just the beginning. Those who also set specific goals with corresponding rewards succeed more quickly, steadily, and enthusiastically. In three months, April lost fourteen inches, ten pounds, and 7 percent body fat. In nine months, Karen lost twenty inches overall, eighteen pounds, and 12 percent body fat. Setting measurable goals and following through with actions and rewards paid off for them, just as it will for you.

Action Goals

As a beginning personal trainer, I didn't help clients set specific goals because they seemed to know what they wanted: to lose weight, tone up, fit into their clothes. We didn't write these goals down with specific action steps because I was afraid that if they didn't reach these goals, they would be more disappointed than if they hadn't set them. For several months, I watched clients who were working out regularly and losing inches and weight become disappointed because they didn't think they were changing fast enough. They focused on what they hadn't achieved instead of what they had. They weren't giving themselves credit for all the work they had done and the progress they had made, and they were becoming frustrated. I began questioning my approach. Maybe my clients should set *specific* goals rather than *general* ones. I decided to try something new with one of my struggling clients, Lisa.

Lisa often came to her workout sessions depressed, angry, disappointed, and pessimistic. She weighed herself twice a week and when she hadn't lost a pound, she felt like a failure. She complained, "I'll never lose this fat. Maybe I should just quit trying. Nothing's happening anyway." Depressed because she wasn't getting the results she wanted, her motivation waned. Lisa was going to quit if we didn't change something, so we created goals with rewards for completing specific actions. Working out five times per week became the goal, not losing weight. She stopped weighing herself so often. Upon completing these actions, she rewarded herself with a predetermined treat of her choice at the end of each week, such as a leisurely bubble bath, relaxing massage, or new clothes.

With this new focus, she felt a sense of accomplishment independent of her weight and appearance. Ironically, when she quit focusing on the results and instead focused on the actions, she began to lose weight and inches. Lisa's success confirmed the necessity for specific, action-based goals.

I began taking this approach with all my clients and they had greater progress and renewed motivation. Writing out their goals and the steps that they were willing to take helped them stay focused.

Slowly, methodically, and safely, they moved toward their goals. When Sara started training, she had never run regularly, but she wanted to run a marathon within twelve months. We divided her goal into twelve month-long segments and began by strengthening her joints and muscles through weight training and jogging for five minutes at a time. Gradually increasing her running time, she was able to run her first 5K race within three months. Within six months, she ran her first half-marathon.

When choosing realistic activities, consider the time required and the amount of time you have. Let's say you want to lose thirty pounds in two months for a class reunion. Even with dieting, you may have to work out two hours per day. Because you don't have the time, your goal may be unrealistic.

My clients sometimes lifted more weight, ran longer, played a sport better, and did more crunches than they thought they could but didn't lose as much weight or as many inches as desired. However, they didn't feel as if they had failed because they had focused on what they *could* control—the *actions*— instead of what they *couldn't*—the *result*s. They knew they were making progress because they were becoming stronger, faster, healthier. If they had made body fat and weight loss their primary goals, these same people would have felt like failures, lost motivation, and stopped working.

During Suzanne's first session, I asked her to think about all the sports and activities she used to love and which ones she'd like to be able to do again. Without hesitation, she said, "Racquetball." And then she laughed because she couldn't imagine playing any time soon. She had been good at the sport before gaining weight. Now she feared embarrassment on the courts. Her six-month goal became playing in a racquetball tournament. She focused on doing the First Steps to Fitness program to the best of her ability, daily, and within a few months, she began playing racquetball again. At six months, she participated in a tournament. The only woman in the finals, Suzanne played the last round against a man half her age and defeated him to win first place.

Although Suzanne surpassed her exercise goal, she didn't fully reach her body weight and fat loss goals, although she had made progress. Because she wasn't completely focused on results, she didn't become disheartened. She stuck with her plan and steadily lost weight and body fat.

Following is a sample Action Goal Chart and then a blank one for you to complete.

ACTION GOALS				
Cardiovascular Goals:	Weekly	Monthly	Quarterly	Yearly
Type of aerobic workout	Run & aerobics class	Run & aerobics class	Run & aerobics class	Run & aerobics class
How many days and how long you will work out	Run 1 mile 4x/week aerobics 1x/week	Run 4x/week, increase 1/2 mile more each month, aerobics 1x/week	Run 3 miles 4x/week aerobics 1x/week	Run 7 miles 3x/week aerobics 1x/week
Other aerobic goals	Try a different aerobic class each week		Complete a 5K race	Complete a 10K race
Strength Goals:				
Type of strength workout	Lift weights	Lift weights	Lift weights	Lift weights
How many days and how long you will work out	2x/week for 25 to 55 minutes	2x/week for 25 to 55 minutes	2x/week for 25 to 55 minutes	2x/week for 25 to 55 minutes
Other strength goals	Follow First Steps to Fitness routine	Follow First Steps to Fitness routine	Follow First Steps to Fitness routine	Follow First Steps to Fitness routine
Flexibility Goals:				
Type of flexibility workout	Stretch at end of each aerobic & weight-lifting workout	Stretch at end of each aerobic & weight-lifting workout, yoga tape	Stretch at end of each aerobic & weight-lifting workout, yoga tape	Stretch at end of each aerobic & weight-lifting workout, yoga tape
How many days and how long you will work out	6x/week after workouts for 10 minutes	6x/week for 10 minutes, yoga tape for 20 min 1x/week	6x/week for 10 minutes, yoga tape for 30 min 1x/week	6x/week for 10 minutes, yoga tape for 40 min 1x/week
Other flexibility goals	Buy yoga tape	Improve leg flexibility		
Diet/Water Goals:				
Type of diet and water goals	64 oz water & 1,500 calories per day, low-glycemic foods	84 oz water & 1,500 calories per day, low-glycemic foods	100 oz water & maintain with 1,600 calories per day	100 oz water & maintain with 1,600 calories per day
How many days you will follow your diet/water plan	6 days a week, 1 day to splurge	6 days a week, 1 day to splurge	6 days a week, 1 day to splurge	6 days a week, 1 day to splurge
Other diet/water goals	Follow First Steps to Fitness program, cut out sweets	Follow First Steps to Fitness program, cut out sweets	Follow First Steps to Fitness program	Follow First Steps to Fitness program
Miscellaneous Goals:				
Other action goals:	Join the new gym in town, strengthen ankles	Enroll in dance class, find a workout partner		

ACTION GOALS				
Cardiovascular Goals:	Weekly	Monthly	Quarterly	Yearly
Type of aerobic workout				
How many days and how long you will work out				
Other aerobic goals				
Strength Goals:				
Type of strength workout				
How many days and how long you will work out				
Other strength goals				
Flexibility Goals:				
Type of flexibility workout				
How many days and how long you will work out				
Other flexibility goals				
Diet/Water Goals:				
Type of diet and water goals				
How many days you will follow your diet/water plan				
Other diet/water goals				
Miscellaneous Goals:				
Other action goals:				

Results Goals

Although you aren't focusing on results goals, it's good to have an idea of how you want to look. The key is to imagine the best while remaining grounded in reality.

How much weight and how many inches can you expect to lose in six months? A year? What is realistic? Let's say we're having a goal-setting meeting and you tell me you want to lose 120 pounds in one year. I would counsel you to consider lowering your goal because you would have to lose two-and-a-half pounds per week. Losing more than one and a half to two pounds per week is unhealthy. To lose more would mean cutting calories so much you would deprive your body of important nutrients and you would also lose valuable muscle, slowing metabolism and making further weight loss difficult. The maximum weight loss in a year would be seventy-five pounds, at one-and-a-half pounds per week. Reaching this goal requires great diligence, commitment, and effort. You should consider whether or not you can perform to the extent that your goals require. Set your goals at a level that causes you to stretch, but not so much that you give up.

Following is a sample Results Goals chart and then a blank one for you to complete.

RESULTS GOALS				
	Weekly	Monthly	Quarterly	Yearly
Weight	Lose 1/2 pound per week	Lose 2 pounds per month	Lose 6 pounds	Lose 24 pounds
Inches/ Measurements	Lose 3/4 inch overall	Lose 3 inches overall	Lose 9 inches overall	Lose 27 inches overall
Body Fat	Lose 1/4% per week	Lose 1% per month	Lose 3% per quarter	Lose 12% in a year
Other		Fit into size 12 jeans	Fit into size 10 jeans	Fit into size 8 jeans

RESULTS GOALS			
	Weekly	Monthly	Quarterly	Yearly
Weight				
Inches/ Measurements				
Body Fat				
Other				

Rewards

Clients who rewarded themselves for accomplishments continued working out despite obstacles. This self-nurturing helped them stay positive and motivated.

Of all my clients, Diana was the best at rewarding herself. While working out, she'd plan her next reward. She would go to a steam room; get a massage; have a nice, juicy, fresh salad; sit in a Jacuzzi.

Another client, Janice, had spent years in sales, winning cruises, trips, and other incentives. Earning rewards was second nature. She would work twice as hard for a reward than she would without one. Splurge Day was her favorite reward—French fries, cheese popcorn, a couple glasses of wine.

Nicky ran every night, and when she returned home rewarded herself with her favorite TV show.

Reward completed actions rather than results. If you set an action goal to run a five-kilometer race and a results goal of losing ten pounds, and you run the race but only lose five pounds, you deserve a reward. You have control over action, not results. If you persist, the results will follow.

What rewards would you enjoy? My clients had different bodies, likes, dislikes, and experiences; therefore, different rewards motivated them. Lisa rewarded herself with quiet time away from the family; Nina bought workout clothes; Janice planned trips; Ann gave herself sweet treats. Rewards don't have to be elaborate or expensive.

Below are some additional ideas:

- **Physical nurturing:** massages, facials, pedicures, manicures
- **Emotional nurturing:** time alone, time with others, time to read, journal, pray, or meditate
- **Experiences:** take a trip, try a new class, begin a hobby, play a sport, go dancing
- **Purchases:** clothes, shoes, exercise equipment, perfume, accessories, books
- **Food/Drink:** special treats, going out to eat, taking the night off from cooking
- **Entertainment:** TV show, movie, play, concert

Jot down rewards you could give yourself. Consider which ones you'd like to work for first.

_____

_____

_____

Some of the most effective rewards are those treats you routinely give yourself. One client splurged on a latte at a coffee shop every day; another bought work-out clothes almost every week; another had a massage every four weeks. The key was to withhold these regular treats until they completed their action goals instead of receiving them automatically. The first client began to have coffee at home throughout the week. At the end of the week, if she'd reached her goals, she treated herself to a latte at one of her favorite coffee shops. The second client bought workout clothes only after she achieved her monthly goals. And the third made her regular massage contingent upon completing her monthly action plan.

Which treats do you routinely give yourself that you could use as rewards? List them here:

_____

_____

_____

Rewards should be appropriate for the amount of effort and commitment required to complete the actions. The more difficult the goal, the greater the reward.

Weekly Rewards

Let's say you followed your workout and eating plan for a week. Your reward might be a new shirt, a new book or tape, an hour nap, a cup of your favorite coffee, or simply Splurge Day.

Monthly Rewards

After a month of good behavior, you deserve a nice reward, one even better than the weekly ones: tickets to the theater, a nice dinner at your favorite restaurant, a new outfit, an hour massage.

Quarterly Rewards

Give yourself something exciting after three months of committed action—a weekend getaway, a day at a spa, a new piece of exercise equipment, a weekend spiritual retreat.

Annual Rewards

Indulge in that reward you've been working for all year—a vacation, a new wardrobe, a week at a spa, a membership at a club you've wanted to join, a new toy.

Write your goals and rewards onto the blank Schedule Sheet that follows the example schedule on the next two pages under the appropriate headings. This will allow you to see everything at a glance. Check the box next to the goals you achieve and the rewards you earn.

SCHEDULE SHEET

WEEK		MON.	TUES.	WED.	THURS.	FRI.	SAT.	SUN.	Weekly Goals		Weekly Rewards	
WEEK 1	WORK-OUT TYPE	Weights Upper Body		Weights Lower Body	Cardio	Cardio	Cardio	Rest Day	run 1 mile 4x ✓ 1 aerobics class ✓ lift weights 2x ✓		new T-shirt	✓
	MEAL PLAN	5 meals 1400 calories	5 meals 1400 calories	5 meals 1400 calories	5 meals 1400 calories	5 meals 1400 calories	Splurge Day	5 meals 1400 calories	64 oz. water daily ✓			
WEEK 2	WORK-OUT TYPE	Weights Upper Body		Weights Lower Body	Cardio	Cardio	Cardio	Rest Day	run 1 1/8 mile 4x ✓ 1 aerobics class ✓ lift weights 2x ✓		a large café latte	✓
	MEAL PLAN	5 meals 1400 calories	5 meals 1400 calories	5 meals 1400 calories	5 meals 1400 calories	5 meals 1400 calories	Splurge Day	5 meals 1400 calories	64 oz. water daily ✓			

SCHEDULE SHEET

WEEK		MON.	TUES.	WED.	THURS.	FRI.	SAT.	SUN.	Weekly Goals		Weekly Rewards	
WEEK 3	WORK-OUT TYPE	Weights Upper Body	Cardio	Weights Lower Body	Cardio	Cardio	Cardio	Rest Day	run 1 1/4 mile 4x ✓ 1 aerobics class ✓ lift weights 2x ✓		massage ✓	
	MEAL PLAN	5 meals 1400 calories	5 meals 1400 calories	5 meals 1400 calories	5 meals 1400 calories	5 meals 1400 calories	Splurge Day	5 meals 1400 calories	64 oz. water daily ✓			
WEEK 4	WORK-OUT TYPE	Weights Upper Body		Weights Lower Body	Cardio	Cardio	Cardio	Rest Day	run 1 1/2 mile 4x ✓ 1 aerobics class ✓ lift weights 2x ✓		time alone ✓	
	MEAL PLAN	4-5 meals 1400 calories	4-5 meals 1400 calories	4-5 meals 1400 calories	4-5 meals 1400 calories	4-5 meals 1400 calories	Splurge Day	4-5 meals 1400 calories	64 oz. water daily ✓			

Monthly Goals:
Increase run by 1/2 mile. Enroll in dance class. Find a workout partner.

Quarterly Goals:
Run a 5K race. Do yoga 5x per week.

Annual Goals:
Run a 10K race. Look into teaching yoga classes.

Monthly Rewards:
Concert Tickets

Quarterly Rewards:
Night's stay at a bed & breakfast.

Annual Rewards:
A five-day cruise.

SCHEDULE SHEET										
WEEK		MON.	TUES.	WED.	THURS.	FRI.	SAT.	SUN.	Weekly Goals	Weekly Rewards
WEEK 1	WORK-OUT TYPE									
	MEAL PLAN									
WEEK 2	WORK-OUT TYPE									
	MEAL PLAN									

SCHEDULE SHEET

WEEK		MON.	TUES.	WED.	THURS.	FRI.	SAT.	SUN.	Weekly Goals	Weekly Rewards
WEEK 3	WORK-OUT TYPE									
	MEAL PLAN									
WEEK 4	WORK-OUT TYPE									
	MEAL PLAN									

Monthly Goals:	Quarterly Goals:	Annual Goals:
Monthly Rewards:	Quarterly Rewards:	Annual Rewards:

Blocks

The following is a list of common mental blocks experienced when attempting to use a rewards system. Put a check next to those that apply to you:

- Guilt about giving yourself rewards
- Fear others will judge you as being selfish or will in some way disapprove
- Unaccustomed to treating yourself kindly
- Unworthiness
- Unable to wait for rewards—give yourself what you want, when you want it
- Ungrateful for rewards
- Laziness about keeping track of actions and rewards

Let's discuss some of these blocks. Maybe you're not used to rewarding yourself. That's okay. We're creatures of habit, so with practice we can make positive thoughts and behaviors our habits.

Perhaps you don't want to wait to complete the actions to get the rewards. You could ask someone to give you your reward after you've earned it. Perhaps there is a dress for sale at a local store. You buy the dress and give it to a friend to hold until you have done what you set out to do. You tell her what you're doing and why. She agrees to help, encourages you, and when you reach your goal, she hands over the dress with a smile.

Others often help us if we ask. For her reward, one client wanted an hour alone in her house to take a bath, sip a glass of wine, and relax in peace and quiet. She told her husband that this was what she wanted for completing her weekly workout and diet plan. Wanting to help her succeed, he took their two children away from the house for more than an hour so she could have her reward.

Another obstacle can be laziness about keeping track of goals, workouts, diet, and rewards. By filling in your Daily Schedule, you hold yourself accountable for the actions you have done, which is extremely important in developing any positive habit. Also, you are reminded to reward your efforts.

Rewarding yourself for correct actions can motivate you to continue. Using a rewards program successfully requires willingness, practice, and consistency.

Care for yourself as much as you care for others. Invest in the moment instead of the outcome. Reward yourself for correct actions. You deserve it.

Goal Collage

The Goal Collage is one of the best motivational exercises I have found. My clients love it. It helps them focus, reminds them of the actions they need to do daily and weekly, and supplies them visual goals to work toward.

If you can visualize, you can actualize. If you can't visualize, it's like trying to find your way out of a forest without a compass or a map. You might eventually find your way, but it may take you much longer, if you get there at all. You may think this exercise is silly and may not want anyone to see what you have made. That's okay. Do it anyway.

Create a positive image of yourself as you *want* to be so that you *can* be. You wouldn't build a house without a blueprint. Psychologist Dr. Joyce Brothers said, "We can't act in a way that is contrary to the way we see ourselves." If you can imagine yourself as fit, buff, hot, energetic, playful, or whatever you desire, then you can act in a way consistent with these images.

To help you envision specifically what you are working toward, create a dream/goals collage. Find several fitness/health or other magazines and clip out photos of people who have what you want or clip out words that inspire you. Maybe you like her midsection, and someone else's legs. Perhaps at one time you were in great shape and you want to look like that again. Find photos of yourself at that time.

Paste these images on a poster board or construction paper. Leave a margin to write your action goals. When you are finished, display your collage on the refrigerator, on your mirror, in front of your treadmill, or anywhere you will see it often.

Just like each of us, this collage is a work in progress. You may find new inspirational photos or quotes you'd like to add. Or perhaps your schedule changes and therefore you need to revamp your workout plan. Also you may find, as did some of my clients, that you'd like to make more than one—a collage for the workout room, one for the refrigerator, another for the bedroom mirror.

Attitude
One part at a time, one day at a time,
we can accomplish any goal we set for ourselves.
Today, I will do one small task that will contribute
toward the achievement of a life goal.
— *Hazelden Foundation*

Check-In

1. On a scale of one to ten, ten being highly positive, how is your attitude?

2. Have you been using the workout and eating-plan worksheets?

chapter nine

Fit Thinking

Now that you've gotten in touch with your innermost desires and have visualized having those things, you will harness the power of thinking to help you get what you want. You have been following the workout and eating plan, striving for goals and rewards, and achieving success. You have been constructing your dream house on the strong foundation you built. But with this dream house, as with most homes, there is continual maintenance to be done. The same is true about mental and emotional states along the fitness path.

Even though you dealt with many issues in the first three chapters, at times negativity may creep in and slow or halt your progress. You may become doubtful, impatient, frustrated, critical. To remain positive, exercise not only your body but also your mind.

As a trainer and an exerciser myself, I've noticed common recurring negative thoughts that hamper fitness progress. The first one we'll discuss is focusing on the "pain" of working out.

Doris, a client, couldn't stay on the bike for more than ten minutes unless she was distracted by someone talking to her or by reading or watching TV. If she wasn't distracted, all she could think about was how much her legs hurt, how bored she was, or how much she wished she were at home eating dinner. Yet, she needed to lose weight. In order to do so, she had to have pleasant distractions while exercising. Psychologists call this dissociation—dissociating the mind from bodily discomfort. Interesting scenery, music, television, and reading material all work well.

Other common roadblocks to fitness progress are focusing on what we haven't achieved instead of what we have and comparing ourselves negatively to others. After three months of following the First Steps to Fitness plan, Sonia had lost seven pounds and twelve inches, but she wasn't satisfied. She complained about her midsection even though she had lost three inches there. She disliked her legs even though she admitted she could see more definition. She wasn't happy with her back because she wanted it to be more muscular.

She also compared herself negatively to others. While training, she would point out others' physical attributes and complain that she could never look like them. She focused on what she didn't have instead of what she did. She became disheartened, discouraged, and depressed—*even though she was making progress!*

Finally, I pointed out how focusing on the negative and comparing herself to others was slowing her progress and suggested she set a goal to stop thinking and saying negative things about herself. She agreed to try. For several weeks, it took much effort for her to turn off the negative thoughts that had been part of her thinking for so long. Every time she would begin to criticize herself, she'd stop and say something encouraging and complimentary instead. Over time, her persistence paid off. Feeling more positive and better about herself, she discovered a newfound enthusiasm for working out and eating right.

Impatience is another common obstacle. We often want results fast and give up if we don't get them in a certain time frame. In the first three weeks of working the program, Beth lost an incredible eight inches. But instead of being happy she lost more than others usually do, she touched her outer thighs and buttocks and said, "Look at this! This fat is still here. I have to do more." Because of her impatience, she began taking pills to increase her metabolism, but they increased her heart rate, kept her awake at night, and made her uncomfortable. After two weeks of taking pills, she hadn't lost any more inches so she stopped and began working the First Steps to Fitness program again. Within four months, she reached her results goals.

Not only are there common obstacles, there are also common solutions. One thought at a time, you can rein in negative thoughts and train your brain to think positively. You are not a victim of your mind unless you choose to be.

Filter your thoughts.
You may catch yourself thinking things such as:
- "Yeah, I've lost a couple of pounds, but I still look like crap. I'll never look much better than this."
- "Working out is too hard. I just don't think I can keep it up. Isn't there an easier way?"

- "I'll always be fat."
- "I'll never amount to anything."
- "No one cares if I feel better about myself or not."
- "I don't care what happens to me."

Judging yourself or getting angry with yourself when you have these thoughts worsens the situation. You can't control the first thought. It's a pattern that has been cultivated for years. It's impulsive and reactive, not logical or productive.

Recognize negative thoughts and replace them with positive ones.

This is difficult, but it gets easier with practice. One trick is to use replacement thoughts that you can buy into at least half way. Otherwise, you'll reject them and the negativity cycle will start all over again. You may find you have to stop your thoughts one hundred times a day at first, but persistence will diminish them. Criticism will become foreign. Compliments and encouragement will become the norm.

Let's say you catch yourself thinking something negative such as, "My legs don't look any different than before I started working out three months ago. Why continue if nothing is going to change?" You realize you need to replace this thought with something better. The following is a list of three potential replacement statements you could use:

1. My legs look good today.
2. I am in the process of toning my body.
3. Because I am patient, hardworking, and committed, I am achieving my goal of nice legs and a fit body.

When you read these statements, what was your reaction? Did you have difficulty believing any of them? Perhaps you couldn't buy into the first statement but you could accept number two or three, at least partially.

The following template can be used to design replacements for negative thoughts. Simply insert the appropriate words.

Positive Replacement Template

I _____ today.

I am in the process of _____ today.

Because I am patient, hardworking, and committed, I am

_____.

Strike the word "want" from your vocabulary.

When you say, "I want," you are actually pushing away what you want. Stating "I want" is a declaration that you don't have something. As a result, you will continue to want as long as you consider yourself lacking. Whereas, stating, "I am," or "I have," even if you are not or do not yet have, opens you up to receive.

Begin training your mind.

List those things that you want, only write them in present tense, stating, "I am" or "I have," before each item. Here are examples:

- I am consistent in my workouts and in my diet.
- I am healthy.
- I am confident in my body.
- I feel sexy.
- I am firm, muscular, and fit.
- I see progress.
- I have a lean but shapely body.
- I have definition in my legs.

Fill in the blanks with your positive affirmations:

I _____.
I _____.
I _____.
I _____.
I _____.
I _____.

I _____ .
I _____ .
I _____ .
I _____ .
I _____ .
I _____ .
I _____ .

Read each of the above affirmations aloud while looking at yourself in a mirror. Do this at least once a day. Add to the list as you please.

Another activity for staying positive and motivated is writing gratitude lists. Jot down everything you have to be grateful for, whether it is your left ear lobe, flat tummy, nice lips, strong arms, your spouse, child, pet, car, and so on:

_____
_____
_____
_____
_____
_____
_____
_____

A gratitude list allows you to focus on what you have instead of what you do not. Create these lists daily or whenever you need your spirits lifted.

With persistence, you can sustain a positive outlook, maintain the dream house you've built, and move forward.

Check-In

1. Where is your gratitude level, on a scale of one to ten, ten being the highest?

2. How many days this week did you follow the First Steps to Fitness program? Is it becoming easier?

chapter ten

Relapse Prevention

At times you may set goals—work out five times per week, lift this much weight, run this far—only to have obstacles get in the way. Life happens: injuries, illness, vacations, family, work, holidays. Some obstacles may be out of your immediate control; others may be within your power to change. Rigidity leads to disappointment. Sometimes you'll have to change plans and goals to fit your life. As Mother Teresa taught, "Don't let what you can't do keep you from doing what you can." No matter the situation, you can always do something positive, even if it's simply drinking lots of water or doing abdominal crunches. Something is better than nothing.

Many clients went through temporary setbacks/relapses. Some of the relapses were self-induced; others were just part of life. They all learned a great deal from the experiences about themselves, their bodies, and their commitment. Often, they emerged from relapse situations with a clearer idea of what to change about their fitness programs. They returned with new energy, enthusiasm, and gratitude. Each relapse is an opportunity to reach a plain where you can catch your breath and thoroughly scan the flat land before deciding which mountain to conquer next.

My client Carrie visited family for the holidays with great plans to work out for the three weeks she was there. But due to family obligations, she didn't have time. Angry and depressed that she hadn't exercised or eaten healthfully, she returned home and had difficulty resuming her normal fitness routine. After several days, Carrie recognized what she was feeling and why. We discussed the importance of remaining flexible so guilt and depression wouldn't overcome her again.

Sara, a client, had been working out religiously for seven months when she found herself doubled over in pain one weekend. She was rushed into the emergency room and then quickly into surgery. The doctors removed an ovarian cyst and told her she couldn't exercise for a month or longer.

She was terrified of losing the progress she had made and losing her motivation. But her fitness lifestyle had become such a part of her life that she could never comfortably go back to being a couch potato. She agonized over the setback until she stopped focusing on what she couldn't change and instead, focused on what she could. She could drink plenty of water, have fewer calories, read diet and exercise books, and let her body heal itself.

A month later, she returned to the gym with a new determination and commitment, ready to make diet and workout changes she hadn't been willing to make before.

What is most likely to derail a fitness program? Stress. It's the number-one predictor of relapse from any behavior change. Stress is defined in the Merriam-Webster's dictionary as "mental, emotional, or physical tension, strain, or distress." Have you ever eaten a whole box of cookies because you were worried or excited? Have you ever become ill around the same time as a stressful event in your life? Almost every fitness magazine includes articles about the negative effects of stress:

- Stress and overeating
- Stress and physical problems
- Stress and fatigue
- Stress and depression and lack of will
- Stress and obesity
- Stress and illness

If added stress can cause us to become ill, to eat more than we need, and to become depressed and lethargic, then stress has tremendous potential to impede our fitness progress.

What causes stress? The Schedule of Recent Experience, a questionnaire used by therapists, lists the most stressful events in our lives. Below are the top ten. Mark the ones you have experienced and jot down when these events occurred.

Event	When Event Occurred
Death of spouse	
Divorce	
Marital separation from mate	
Detention in jail or institution	
Death of a close family member	
Major personal injury or illness	
Marital problems	
Being fired at work	
Marital reconciliation with mate	
Retirement from work	

How many have you gone through in the last year, the last six months, the last month?

According to the Symptoms of Stress Continuum, another therapeutic tool, we experience stress symptoms along a continuum that begins with physical manifestations. If the stress goes unchecked, it can lead to mental, emotional, social, and spiritual problems.

Have you recently experienced any of the following stress symptoms?

- **Physical:** fatigue, sleeping problems, abuse of alcohol or drugs, more accidents, over- or undereating, increased minor illnesses, sexual problems

- **Mental:** concentration difficulty, increased mistakes, forgetfulness, poor performance, lack of enthusiasm
- **Emotional:** lower self-image, depression, cynicism/negativity, vague feelings of distress, fear, anxiety, inability to slow down, irritability, insensitivity to others
- **Social:** withdrawal from others, breakdown in communication, complaining, decreased trust in others, compromised values, reluctance to share, decreased ability to problem-solve
- **Spiritual**: hopelessness, doubtfulness about the existence of a Higher Power, loneliness, pervading sense of sadness, difficulty seeing the positive in life, thoughts about ending your life, disenchantment

Where are you along this continuum?

When you're stressed, your body produces high levels of the stress hormone cortisol. Your body interprets this surge in cortisol as a need for energy, such as that in food, leading to binges or excessive snacking.

You can avoid or minimize stress. A study in *Integrative Physiological and Behavior Science* (April-June 1998) showed a 23 percent reduction in cortisol levels through emotional self-management techniques such as meditation and controlled breathing. Also, exercise and proper diet help alleviate stress. An article in *Fitness Management* magazine stated that, "Reduction in anxiety and mood improvements have been reported to continue for at least thirty minutes and perhaps as long as six hours after an exercise bout has ceased."

The following are additional stress relievers:
- Eat at least one balanced hot meal per day
- Get seven or eight hours of sleep at least four times per week
- Give and receive affection regularly
- Drink fewer than five alcoholic drinks per week
- Attend social or club activities
- Do something fun at least once per week
- Drink fewer than three cups of caffeinated beverages per day
- Take quiet time for yourself during the day
- Develop a network of friends and acquaintances

Factors that affect fitness adherence can be external or internal, and they can be in your control or out of your control. The following are potential relapse situations, grouped accordingly:

External factors/Not in your control:

Physical limitations (injuries, disabilities, illnesses, surgeries): You have to heal before continuing your routine, or perhaps you're limited to certain exercises. (Challenge: Could you have prevented the physical limitation? What could you learn from this experience?)

Holidays/Vacations: Staying under someone else's roof, you may not have complete control over your plans. Perhaps you're served foods you don't normally eat. (Challenge: Are you okay with being "different" by eating healthy foods or by working out when others around you choose not to?)

Work/Family obligations: On days you are overtasked—work deadlines, family responsibilities, errands—you try to make time for yourself but often have more immediate issues to contend with. It's difficult to squeak in workouts and healthy eating. (Challenge: Can you better plan your weeks and days to create more time for yourself? Are you taking on responsibilities you don't need? Make a list of your priorities. Are you using a busy life as an excuse?)

Internal factors/Not in your control:

Clinical depression or moderate depression/grief: A depressed emotional state makes performing normal activities difficult. Some situations require professional guidance. (Challenge: Emotional states improve from working out, so don't wait to "be in the mood." Go for a walk, dance to your favorite tunes, swim in a nice, warm pool. Notice how your mood changes.)

External factors/Within your control:

Make good choices: The kinds of food you have in the house, restaurants you frequent, exercises you perform (those less likely to cause injury). (Challenge: What foods do you have in the house that are difficult to stop eating once you start? Do you need to have these foods around?)

Plan ahead: When traveling, whenever possible, choose hotels with exercise rooms, find a gym in the area, make physical activity (such as walks and hikes) part of your daily life. Take lightweight, portable exercise equipment with you, such as bands, tubes, water dumbbells, and videotapes. Or do a routine using only your body as resistance and items in your room: lunges holding onto a chair, abdominal crunches, tricep dips off of a bed or a chair, push-ups. (Challenge: What will you do on your next trip to stay fit?)

Be prepared: Carry food in your car, purse, suitcase. (Challenge: What kinds of foods could you take with you?)

Internal factors/Within your control

Your thoughts, attitudes, and feelings: To some extent, you can change all three. If you think bad thoughts about yourself, you're going to feel bad. We are what we think we are. (Challenge: For one day, write down all the negative thoughts you have about yourself and how you feel as a result. For one day, try to think positive things about yourself all day and write down how you feel.)

Don't give away your power: If you're trying to please someone, you're giving him or her your power. If you're bending your life around an unrealistic ideal, you're giving your power up to that ideal. Instead, keep your power. (Challenge: To whom or to what have you been giving your power today?)

How do you come back from a relapse? Here are the seven steps:

1. Recognize that you've had a setback.
2. Admit it to yourself and to another, if you'd like.
3. Forgive yourself.
4. Recommit to your program—this process is life-long, not short-term.
5. Practice mental fitness to keep a positive outlook.
6. Return to working out and eating healthy as soon as possible.
7. Seek help from a health or fitness professional, friend, or mentor, if needed.

Identify and accept those things you can change and those you cannot. Then start changing those things that you can.

The Serenity Prayer sums up this idea well:

God, grant me the Serenity to accept the things I cannot change,
Courage to change the things I can
And Wisdom to know the difference.

I wrote my own version to help me with my body image and fitness:
God, grant me the Serenity to accept the things I cannot
change without cosmetic surgery,
The Courage to change the things I can without killing myself trying,
And the Wisdom to know the difference between supermodels and real women.

Challenge: Design your own Serenity Prayer

Those dark days when going to the gym seems as impossible and as unlikely as running for President, or when standing in the grocery store, you swear that gigantic chocolate chip cookie leapt into your cart, what do you do? Continue on. Go back through this book and reread the chapters that deal with whatever roadblocks you're experiencing. Or call a friend who is a fitness enthusiast and borrow her enthusiasm until yours returns. And always remember that you don't have to do this perfectly. Just make a stab at it and do the best you can every day.

Attitude

"The longer I live, the more I realize the
impact of attitude on life.
Attitude is more important than the past,
than education, than money, than circumstances.
It is more important than failures, than successes,
Than what other people think, say or do.
It is more important than
appearance, giftedness, or skill.
It will make or break a company, a home.
The remarkable thing is you have a choice every day regarding the
Attitude you will embrace for that day.
We cannot change our past…
We cannot change the fact that people
Will act in a certain way.
We cannot change the inevitable.
The only thing we can do is play on the
One string we have, and that is our attitude.

I am convinced that life is ten percent what
Happens to me and ninety percent how I react to it.
And so it is with you."
— *Author Unknown*

Check-In

1. Where is your stress level today on a scale of one to ten, ten being the highest?

2. Have you reached your goals this week and received your rewards?

3. Have you had any of your favorite foods on your Splurge Day?

chapter eleven

Fitness Fellowship

Our deepest fear is not that we are inadequate.
Our deepest fear is that we are powerful beyond measure.
It is our Light, not our Darkness, that most frightens us.
We ask ourselves, Who am I to be brilliant, gorgeous, talented, fabulous?
Actually, who are you not to be? You are a child of God.
Your playing small does not serve the World.
There is nothing enlightening about shrinking so that other people
Won't feel unsure around you.
We were born to make manifest the Glory of God that is within us.
It is not just in some of us; it is in everyone.
As we let our own Light shine, we unconsciously give other people
Permission to do the same.
As we are liberated from our own fear, our presence automatically
Liberates others.
— *Nelson Mandela, Inaugural Speech, 1994*

You have done something extraordinary and unique. You have faced and worked through any thoughts and feelings that may have kept you stuck. You have proven that you have power and that you are not a victim. By making good choices and following through with plans, you've steadily succeeded in improving your fitness.

What if you shared with everyone what you've found? There would be fewer stress-related illnesses, cases of depression, and premature deaths and more strength, peace, health, and self-esteem.

Following are examples of how people with strong belief and steady action have changed the world.

A group of California women, outraged by the death of a young girl killed by a drunk driver, formed Mothers Against Drunk Driving, or MADD. This driver was actually out on bail from one of several previous arrests when he struck the girl. His penalty? Two years in jail but no time served, only parole and community service. By banding together, the founding women changed laws and penalties and raised awareness. Others shared their conviction and within twenty years MADD grew to include chapters in all fifty states and several other countries.

MADD helped establish the federal minimum drinking age of twenty-one. They helped decrease the percentage of alcohol-related traffic crashes by 20 percent from 1980 to 1997. Through perseverance, these few founding mothers remained focused on their goal and made dramatic positive changes in the world.

In 1986, a visionary gay rights activist, Cleve Jones, and his friends organized the NAMES Project Foundation and began a patchwork quilt of the names of loved ones who had perished from AIDS. Public response was overwhelming—the foundation received quilt panels and supplies from many U.S. cities. The first national tour of the quilt raised nearly $500,000 for AIDS service organizations. By 2000, the quilt grew to 44,000 panels and the tours raised more than three million dollars. This project that started with one man turned into the longest ongoing community arts project in the world.

I am not suggesting we organize MACF, Mothers Against Chubby Families, or produce quilts with names of loved ones who are out of shape. But by taking some simple actions, we can create a fitness revolution and help make the world a better place.

Let Your Light Shine/Be an Example

Others may be noticing the changes in you and wanting what you have. But do you notice them? Sixty percent of adult Americans are overweight and not doing anything consistently about it. Three hundred thousand Americans die each year from obesity-related illnesses, according to The Centers for Disease Control. In this country with plenty of fitness facilities, healthy foods, and information, many people are out of shape and suffering because of it. How many of your friends are unhappy with their appearance? Or in how they feel? You may be the only example they have of how to overcome fitness obstacles.

When people ask, "How did you do it?" and you tell them, "Hard work, dedication, honesty, willingness," they nod their heads as if they're listening. But unless you tell them that a magical potion, technique, or gadget will help them lose weight in twenty-four hours, they tune out. They often don't want to hear the truth until they're willing to change.

However, your success may help them become willing. They start to believe that if you can do it, so can they. They begin to accept that maybe there is no easy way and that maybe the work is worth it.

When Heather began working out, she weighed more than two hundred pounds and was depressed. After just a couple of months of exercising and eating right, she had lost several inches and pounds and her attitude had improved greatly. Except for a few bumps in the road, her progress has been steady ever since. Now her coworkers tell her how proud they are of her and how much she has motivated them to exercise. Heather has been floored by the attention and praise she has received. Her motivation was to lose weight, not inspire other people. She's not always comfortable being in the spotlight or answering people's fitness questions, but she continues caring for herself, thus inspiring others.

Theresa also began at more than two hundred pounds. One of the strongest clients I ever had, she worked extremely hard during our sessions and her strength often amazed people in the gym. She lost weight and inches; however, it wasn't her progress so much that inspired people but her determination and commitment. Unlike Heather, Theresa was not reluctant to be in the spotlight and to lead people to fitness.

Like it or not, your status has been elevated. You've become a role model. People around you will praise you and talk about your success to others. Do you agree with Nelson Mandela's speech that as children of God we were meant to be brilliant, gorgeous, talented, and fabulous?

Gym Camaraderie

Wherever you exercise—the gym, studio, or track—there are people working toward similar goals. Be open to the camaraderie and support of your fellow exercisers. Share workout tips; talk to keep your mind off physical discomfort; encourage, cheer for, and congratulate each other. Be an example to those just beginning their fitness path or those who might be burned out. You'll probably never know how many people miss you when you don't show up to the gym for a while.

I've seen and experienced this camaraderie myself many times. Several years ago, I moved cross-country a few times and joined new gyms and met new people each time. Within a few weeks, the gym members would expect to see me there, and if I missed a few days, they'd ask me where I'd been and if everything was okay. Some of us would talk about work, family, fitness, what works and doesn't work. Being at the gym helped curb my loneliness in a new town where I knew few people. It prevented me from going home right after work to sit on the couch, feel sorry for myself, and eat to make myself feel better.

I've been at the same gym for five years now and have established close friendships with women I have met. We've gone dancing and out to lunch, movies, concerts, and parties. We've helped each other find jobs, change workout programs and diets, evaluate our progress, and more.

Workout Partners

The majority of people prefer to work out in groups rather than alone. If this is true for you, ask someone to be your workout partner. Or gather a group of people you enjoy being around who also want to be fit. Days you don't want to work out, you may go because you want to see your friends or because you said you'd be there.

Many clients' consistency and attitude improved when they partnered up with others as committed to working out as they were. Theresa had several different workout partners. When one couldn't make it, she'd ask another. By making dates to meet them at the gym, she knew she would show up. I would see them at the gym lifting weights and laughing, or on the cardio machines, talking to make the time pass faster. Partnering up worked for Theresa—she lost weight and kept it off.

What if you work out alone at home? I often do. It's quiet, easier to focus, and faster because I don't have to wait to use equipment. But I don't always work out at home alone. On days I want company, I'll invite friends to join me. On days I don't feel motivated, I'll go to the gym because I know I'll work harder with others around me.

Sometimes friends need a little push to start exercising. Perhaps you can ask them to work out with you. Be careful that their presence doesn't hinder your own progress. Most likely, helping another will rejuvenate and inspire you. You'll realize how far you've come. One client, Beverly, began bringing her friend Diana to the gym. Diana was a recent widow who was depressed and thirty pounds overweight. Working out together made Diana smile more and worry less and helped Beverly stay committed.

Fitness Fellowship Groups

Fellowship in and outside the workout facility is key to improving, maintaining, and adhering to a fitness lifestyle. It is also where you can make the greatest impact on others. Because some don't experience camaraderie in their workout facility, others desire more intimate sharing, and still others want a safe environment to work through the First Steps to Fitness book, Fitness Fellowship groups were created. These are discussion groups in which women come together regularly to read *The First Steps to Fitness*, do the assignments, and share ideas and experiences.

How do you become part of a group? First, ask around, call local fitness facilities, or look online to see if one has already been started in your area. If not, invite friends, family, and acquaintances who are interested in becoming more fit to join you in a group. You may want to ask your workout facility to help you promote your group. They may even offer you a place to hold your meetings.

One format that has worked well is for each participant to read and come prepared to discuss a chapter each week. Respect each other's experiences and stories by not repeating what was said in the group to others outside of it. Make this a safe place to learn. Even if you have already worked through the book, you may discover more. You may face different challenges today than you did yesterday. Cultivating a supportive network will help ensure continued progress.

- You are not alone.
- You can help others and yourself more than you ever imagined.
- Your commitment and generosity have a global effect.
- In this way, we lead each other to fuller, happier, healthier lives.
- What an honor it is to be a part of such a revolution.

Check-In

1. How have you changed since beginning this book?
2. How have you positively affected others?
3. What are you most grateful for today?

APPENDIX

Exercise Descriptions

Upper Body

Chest Fly

Target Muscle: Chest

Getting into Position: Sit at the chest fly machine with arms at a ninety-degree angle. Keep your upper arms parallel with the floor.

Completing the Exercise: Start with your elbows in line with your shoulders. Bring your arms together in front of you, keeping your chest held high. Return to the start position, not letting your elbows come back past your shoulders.

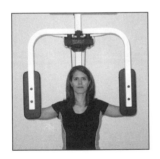 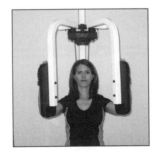 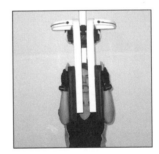

Chest Dumbbell Press

Target Muscle: Chest

Getting into Position: Lay on a bench with your knees bent and feet up to protect your lower back. Hold a dumbbell in each hand.

Completing the Exercise: Begin the exercise with your arms extended straight above you but not locked. Bend your elbows out to the side and bring down until they are in line with your shoulders. To prevent shoulder strain, do not let your elbows come down past your shoulders.

Then push the dumbbells up until your arms are extended again. Keep your chest raised and shoulder blades back throughout the exercise.

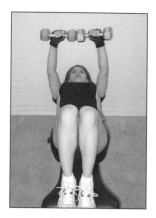 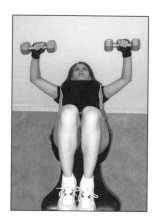

Lat Pull Downs

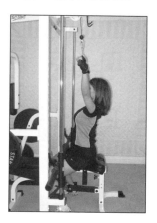

Target Muscle: Upper Back

Getting into Position: Grasp pull-down bar at a wide angle, palms facing forward.

Completing the Exercise: Pull the bar down toward your chest. Keep your chest raised as if a string is attached to your chest and pulling it up toward the ceiling. Lift your chest to meet the bar. Hold for a couple of seconds before raising your arms.

Back Dumbbell Row

Target Muscle: Upper Back

Getting into Position: With one foot on the ground and a dumbbell in the corresponding hand, place the other knee and hand on a bench. Lean over until your back is flat and parallel with the floor.

Completing the Exercise: Let your arm with the dumbbell hang straight while you bring back the shoulder blade. Then bring the arm up, bending the elbow and keeping it close to your side. Hold for a couple of seconds before lowering your arm.

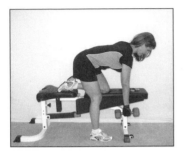 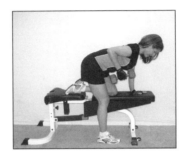

Shoulder Dumbbell Press

Target Muscle: Shoulder

Getting into Position: Stand with feet shoulder-width apart. Hold a dumbbell in each hand at shoulder level, with palms facing forward.

Completing the Exercise: Raise arms straight over your head. Do not lock your elbows or arch your lower back. Then lower the dumbbells back to shoulder level.

Variation: When you raise the dumbbells over your head, bring them together at the top before lowering them.

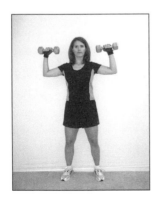 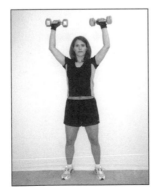

Shoulder Lateral Raise

Target Muscle: Shoulder

Getting into Position: Stand with feet shoulder-width apart and knees slightly bent. Hold weights in your hands, palms facing your sides.

Completing the Exercise: With your arms slightly bent, raise the dumbbells out from your sides and up to level with your shoulders. Then lower back to your sides.

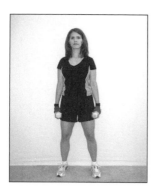 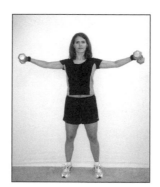

Triceps Press

Target Muscle: Triceps

Getting into Position: Stand up straight with feet shoulder-width apart. Grasp bar with palms down.

Completing the Exercise: Start with the bar pulled down so your arms are at a ninety-degree angle. Keep your elbows in to your sides as you push the bar down to the tops of your thighs, hold for a couple of seconds, and then return to a ninety-degree angle.

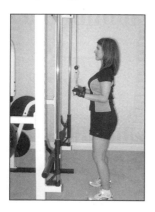 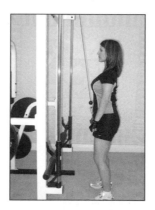

Triceps Dumbbell Extensions

Target Muscle: Triceps

Getting into Position: Stand with feet shoulder-width apart. Hold a dumbbell in one hand and raise that arm over your head. Use the other hand to hold the raised arm next to your head throughout the exercise.

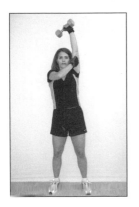 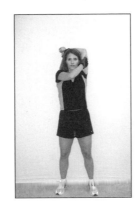

Completing the Exercise: With your palm facing forward, bend the raised arm behind your head and towards the opposite shoulder. Then raise the arm until it is straight up and down again and the elbow is not locked.

Preacher Curls

Target Muscle: Biceps

Getting into Position: Sit at a preacher curl bench. Hold either a bar or dumbbells with palms up, elbows in line with your shoulders, back straight, and chest lifted. You should be sitting high enough so that when you extend your arms down the bench, your elbows touch the bench one-quarter to one-half of the way down without you having to lean over.

Completing the Exercise: Hold the weight in your hands, palms up, at the top of the bench.

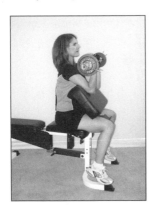 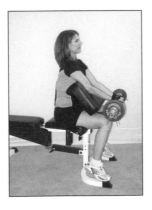

Lower your arms down the bench until your elbows are only slightly bent. Then lift the weight back up to the top. Keep your wrists straight throughout the exercise.

Variation: Do the exercise with dumbbells with your hands facing inward toward each other instead of upward. This position puts less strain on the wrists.

Bicep Hammer Curls

Target Muscle: Biceps

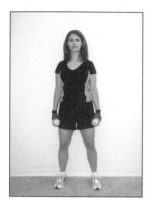 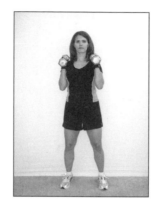

Getting into Position: Stand with feet shoulder-width apart. Hold weights with your palms facing in to your sides.

Completing the Exercise: Start with your arms straight but not locked. Keeping elbows at your sides, bend your arms and bring weights up to the front of your shoulders. Then lower and repeat.

Lower Body

Squats

Target Muscle: Gluteus, Quadriceps, Hamstring

Getting into Position: Your feet are shoulder-width apart. Position the bar so that it rests on the tops of your shoulders. Use a pad on the bar or a towel around your neck to help reduce the pressure of the bar on your neck. Hold on to the bar so that your hands are placed wider than your shoulders and your palms are facing outward. Leaning your shoulders back on the bar, walk your feet out about twelve to fourteen inches.

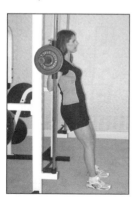 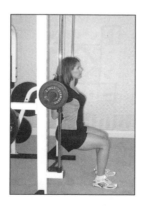

Completing the Exercise: Bring your hips back and bend your knees as if you were sitting in a chair. Your hips should be in line with your shoulders, legs at a ninety-degree angle, and knees directly over or behind your ankles. Then push the bar up as you stand, leaving your feet in the same place, twelve to fourteen inches in front of you.

Lunges with Knee Raise

Target Muscle: Gluteus, Quadriceps, Hamstring

Getting into Position: Stand sideways next to a wall. Place the hand closest to the wall on the wall for support and hold a weight in the other hand. Feet should be shoulder-width apart.

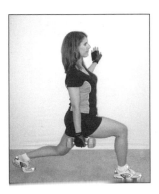

Completing the Exercise: Taking the leg that is closest to the wall, extend it behind you as far as you can. Bend both knees as you lower yourself toward the ground. Your front knee should be directly above or behind your ankle to prevent knee strain. Lower yourself until your front leg is parallel with the ground. Then come back up, bringing that back leg forward and into a knee raise, squeezing the gluteus muscle of the supporting leg as you do so. Do all of your reps on one leg before switching to the other leg.

Variations: When you feel strong enough, do the exercise with a weight in both hands instead of using the wall for support.

Hamstring Curls

Target Muscle: Hamstring

Getting into Position: Lay prone on a hamstring curl bench with your ankles under the bar. Your knees should be aligned with the machine's pivot point. Your hands should be holding onto the bench or other support so your upper back does not lift off of the bench as you bring your legs up.

Completing the Exercise: Bring your feet in toward your glutes without arching your lower back beyond its normal curve.

Variations: Point your toes throughout the exercise to feel the lift more in your calves.

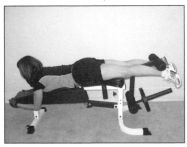 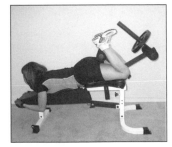

Quadriceps Extensions

Target Muscle: Quadriceps

Getting into Position: Sit up straight on a quadriceps extension machine, knees aligned with the machine's pivot point, toes pointing forward or slightly outward.

Completing the Exercise: Extend your legs. Do not lock your knees. Hold for a couple of seconds before lowering.

Variations: Lift one leg at a time, completing a set of repetitions for one leg before switching to the other leg.

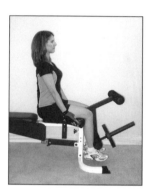 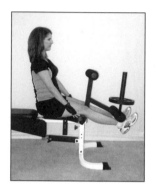

Calf Raise

Target Muscle: Calves

Getting into Position: Stand with feet shoulder-width apart and pointing forward. The bar should rest across the top of the shoulders.

Completing the Exercise: Lift up on to your toes. Come down without letting your heels touch the floor. Keep knees soft but do not bend as you go up and down.

Variations: Turn feet slightly outward. Use dumbbells or weight plates instead of the bar.

Outer Thigh Lift

Target Muscle: Outer Thighs

Getting into Position: Lay on the floor on your side, your hips stacked on top of each other, resting on your elbow. If using weight, hold it on the top leg or use an ankle weight.

Completing the Exercise: Lift the top leg as high as you can while keeping your hips in line with each other. Point your foot downward at an angle and keep your body in a straight line.

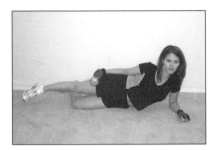
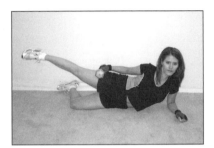

Inner Thigh Lift

Target Muscle: Inner Thighs

Getting into Position: Lay on the floor on your side, leaning back slightly. Bend the top leg and put your foot on the floor. Keep the bottom leg straight with your inner thigh facing up to the ceiling. If you are using weight, hold the weight on top of the bottom thigh or use an ankle weight.

Completing the Exercise: Lift your straight leg as high as you can without leaning forward or backward, keeping your inner thigh facing the ceiling.

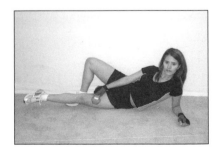
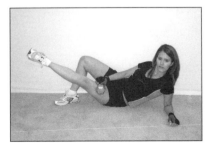

Lower Back Extension on the Ball

Target Muscle: Lower Back

Getting into Position: Lay face down with your hips centered over the top of the ball. Keep your hands behind your head and your legs straight. Place your feet wide for balance.

Completing the Exercise: Simultaneously push hips into the ball and lift upper body. Do not over-arch the lower back.

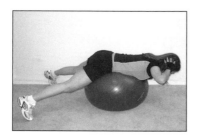 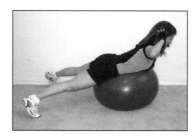

Variations: This exercise can also be done on the floor. Hold a weight behind your head to add difficulty.

Abdominal

Ab Curl on the Bench

Target Muscle: Abdominal

Getting into Position: Lay on the bench with your feet under the bar. Hold knees with your hands until you are ready to begin the exercise.

Completing the Exercise: Hold the outside of your legs as you slowly roll your back down the bench, keeping your back rounded. Go down as far as you feel comfortable without straining your lower back. Then use your abdominal muscles to pull yourself back up.

Variations: Hold a weight on your chest. Rotate your torso to each side before pulling yourself back up (see photo to the right).

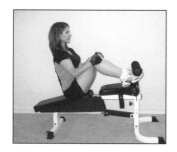 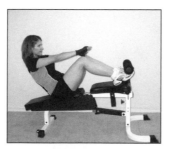 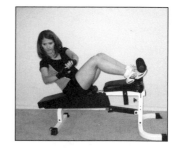

Basic Crunch on the Ball

Target Muscle: Abdominal

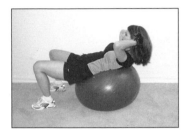

Getting into Position: Lay on the ball, face up, hands behind your head, feet on the ground.

Completing the Exercise: As you lift your upper body off of the ball, push your hips into the ball. Keep chin raised as if you are holding an apple between your chin and your chest. Come up as far as you can, hold for several seconds, and then lower back down.

Crunch on the Floor

Target Muscle: Abdominal

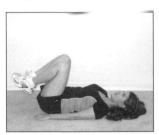

Getting into Position: Lay on the floor with arms by your sides, hands pressed into the floor. Bend knees.

Completing the Exercise: Bring knees up together and lift them toward your chest, lifting your hips off the floor as far as you can without straining the lower back. Then lower your hips until the lower back touches the floor.

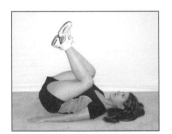

Variations: Instead of leaving your hands on the floor, bring them behind your head and bring your upper body up as you bring your knees toward your chest (see photo to the right). Or, extend the legs instead of keeping them bent throughout the exercise. Try this with or without lifting your upper body off the floor (see photos below).

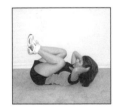

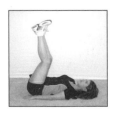
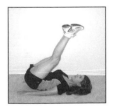
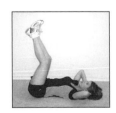
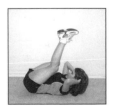

Shoulder-to-Knee Crunch on the Ball

Target Muscle: Abdominal

Getting into Position: Lay face up on the ball. The higher on the ball your lower body rests, the greater the difficulty. Place one hand on the wall or other support and the other behind your head.

Completing the Exercise: Extend the leg closest to the wall, leaving the other foot planted on the ground. Bring together the knee and opposite shoulder. Then lower the leg without letting the foot touch the ground before doing the next repetition.

Variation: Hold a weight on the shoulder that you are lifting to add difficulty.

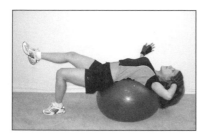 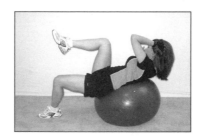

Dumbbell Side Crunch

Target Muscle: Abdominal/Side

Getting into Position: Stand with feet shoulder-width apart and knees slightly bent. Hold a dumbbell in one hand and put the other hand behind your head.

Completing the Exercise: Lean to the side in which you are holding the dumbbell. Lean as far as you can without bending your knees more or twisting your torso. Then return to standing straight.

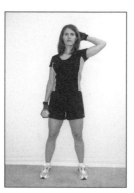 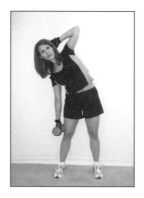

Charts

TARGET HEART RATE CHART

	220	This number is the maximum heart rate of a child at birth
Minus		Your age
Equals		Your maximum heart rate
Times	.70	Appropriate intensity level
Equals		Your target heart rate

FIRST STEPS TO FITNESS AEROBIC PROGRAM

Before working out, how do I feel emotionally? Physically?

Planned Program

Date:	Activity:	Time:
Warm Up:		5 minutes
Main Section:		15–35 min.
Cool Down:		5 minutes
Total Time:		25–45 min.

FIRST STEPS TO FITNESS AEROBIC PROGRAM

Completed Program

Date:	Activity:	Time:
Warm Up:		
Main Section:		
Cool Down:		
Total Time:		

After working out, how do I feel emotionally?
Physically?

FIRST STEPS TO FITNESS RESISTANCE PROGRAM
Week One Upper Body

Before I start, how do I feel physically? Emotionally?

Planned Program

Date:

Warm up:

	Formula for Amount of Weight	Weight	Reps	Seconds Between Sets
Chest Exercise	12-Rep Max Weight		10-12	60
_____	Same		10-12	0
Back Exercise	12-Rep Max Weight		10-12	60
_____	Same		10-12	0
Shoulder Exercise	12-Rep Max Weight		10-12	60
_____	Same		10-12	0
Tricep Exercise	12-Rep Max Weight		10-12	60
_____	Same		10-12	0
Bicep Exercise	12-Rep Max Weight		10-12	60
_____	Same		10-12	0
Abdominal Exercise	12-Rep Max Weight		10-12	60
_____	Same		10-12	0

Stretches (Put a check when complete):

Chest	✓
Back	✓
Shoulder	✓
Tricep	✓
Bicep	✓
Abdominal	✓
Total Workout Time:	28 minutes

Completed Program			
Date:			
Warm up:			
	Weight	Reps	Seconds Between Sets
Chest Exercise _____			
Back Exercise _____			
Shoulder Exercise _____			
Tricep Exercise _____			
Bicep Exercise _____			
Abdominal Exercise _____			

Stretches (Put a check when complete):	
Chest	
Back	
Shoulder	
Tricep	
Bicep	
Abdominal	
Total Workout Time:	

After working out, how do I feel emotionally? Physically?

FIRST STEPS TO FITNESS RESISTANCE PROGRAM
Week One Lower Body

Before I start, how do I feel physically? Emotionally?

	Planned Program			
Date:		Warm up:		
	Formula for Amount of Weight	Weight	Reps	Seconds Between Sets
Glute Exercise _____	12-Rep Max Weight		10-12	60
	Same		10-12	0
Quadricep Exercise _____	12-Rep Max Weight		10-12	60
	Same		10-12	0
Hamstring Exercise _____	12-Rep Max Weight		10-12	60
	Same		10-12	0
Inner Thigh Exercise _____	12-Rep Max Weight		10-12	60
	Same		10-12	0
Outer Thigh Exercise _____	12-Rep Max Weight		10-12	60
	Same		10-12	0
Calf Exercise _____	12-Rep Max Weight		10-12	60
	Same		10-12	0
Abdominal Exercise _____	12-Rep Max Weight		10-12	60
	Same		10-12	0
Lower Back Exercise _____	12-Rep Max Weight		10-12	60
	Same		10-12	0

Stretches (Put a check when complete):	
Glute	√
Quadricep	√
Hamstring	√
Inner & Outer Thigh	√
Calf	√
Abdominal & Lower Back	√
Total Workout Time:	28 minutes

Completed Program			
Date:			
Warm up:			
	Weight	Reps	Seconds Between Sets
Glute Exercise _____			
Quadricep Exercise _____			
Hamstring Exercise _____			
Inner Thigh Exercise _____			
Outer Thigh Exercise _____			
Calf Exercise _____			
Abdominal Exercise _____			
Lower Back Exercise _____			

Stretches (Put a check when complete):

Glute	
Quadricep	
Hamstring	
Inner & Outer Thigh	
Calf	
Abdominal & Lower Back	
Total Workout Time:	

After working out, how do I feel emotionally? Physically?

FIRST STEPS TO FITNESS RESISTANCE PROGRAM
Week Two Upper Body

Before I start, how do I feel physically? Emotionally?

	Planned Program			
Date:		Warm up:		
	Formula for Amount of Weight	Weight	Reps	Seconds Between Sets
Chest Exercise	12-Rep Max Weight plus 5-10 lb.		8-10	60
	Same		8-10	60
_____	Same		8-10	0
Back Exercise	12-Rep Max Weight plus 5-10 lb.		8-10	60
	Same		8-10	60
_____	Same		8-10	0
Shoulder Exercise	12-Rep Max Weight plus 5-10 lb.		8-10	60
	Same		8-10	60
_____	Same		8-10	0
Tricep Exercise	12-Rep Max Weight plus 5-10 lb.		8-10	60
	Same		8-10	60
_____	Same		8-10	0
Bicep Exercise	12-Rep Max Weight plus 5-10 lb.		8-10	60
	Same		8-10	60
_____	Same		8-10	0
Abdominal Exercise	12-Rep Max Weight plus 5-10 lb.		8-10	60
	Same		8-10	60
_____	Same		8-10	0

Stretches (Put a check when complete):	
Chest	√
Back	√
Shoulder	√
Tricep	√
Bicep	√
Abdominal	√
Total Workout Time:	36 minutes

Completed Program			
Date:			
Warm up:			
	Weight	Reps	Seconds Between Sets
Chest Exercise _____			
Back Exercise _____			
Shoulder Exercise _____			
Tricep Exercise _____			
Bicep Exercise _____			
Abdominal Exercise _____			

Stretches (Put a check when complete):	
Chest	
Back	
Shoulder	
Tricep	
Bicep	
Abdominal	
Total Workout Time:	

After working out, how do I feel emotionally? Physically?

FIRST STEPS TO FITNESS RESISTANCE PROGRAM
Week Two Lower Body

Before I start, how do I feel physically? Emotionally?

	Planned Program			
Date:		Warm up:		
	Formula for Amount of Weight	Weight	Reps	Seconds Between Sets
Glute Exercise	12-Rep Max Weight plus 5-10 lb.		8-10	60
	Same		8-10	60
_____	Same		8-10	0
Quadricep Exercise	12-Rep Max Weight plus 5-10 lb.		8-10	60
	Same		8-10	60
_____	Same		8-10	0
Hamstring Exercise	12-Rep Max Weight plus 5-10 lb.		8-10	60
	Same		8-10	60
_____	Same		8-10	0
Inner Thigh Exercise	12-Rep Max Weight plus 5-10 lb.		8-10	60
	Same		8-10	60
_____	Same		8-10	0
Outer Thigh Exercise	12-Rep Max Weight plus 5-10 lb.		8-10	60
	Same		8-10	60
_____	Same		8-10	0
Calf Exercise	12-Rep Max Weight plus 5-10 lb.		8-10	60
	Same		8-10	60
_____	Same		8-10	0
Abdominal Exercise	12-Rep Max Weight plus 5-10 lb.		8-10	60
	Same		8-10	60
_____	Same		8-10	0
Lower Back Exercise	12-Rep Max Weight plus 5-10 lb.		8-10	60
	Same		8-10	60
_____	Same		8-10	0

Stretches (Put a check when complete):

Glute	√
Quadricep	√
Hamstring	√
Inner & Outer Thigh	√
Calf	√
Abdominal & Lower Back	√
Total Workout Time:	36 minutes

Completed Program			
Date:			
Warm up:			
	Weight	Reps	Seconds Between Sets
Glute Exercise _____			
Quadricep Exercise _____			
Hamstring Exercise _____			
Inner Thigh Exercise _____			
Outer Thigh Exercise _____			
Calf Exercise _____			
Abdominal Exercise _____			
Lower Back Exercise _____			

Stretches (Put a check when complete):	
Glute	
Quadricep	
Hamstring	
Inner & Outer Thigh	
Calf	
Abdominal & Lower Back	
Total Workout Time:	

After working out, how do I feel emotionally? Physically?

FIRST STEPS TO FITNESS RESISTANCE PROGRAM
Week Three Upper Body

Before I start, how do I feel physically? Emotionally?

Planned Program

Date:		Warm up:		
	Formula for Amount of Weight	Weight	Reps	Seconds Between Sets
Chest Exercise	12-Rep Max Weight plus 10-15 lb.		6-8	60
	Same		6-8	60
	Same		6-8	60
_____	Same		6-8	0
Back Exercise	12-Rep Max Weight plus 10-15 lb.		6-8	60
	Same		6-8	60
	Same		6-8	60
_____	Same		6-8	0
Shoulder Exercise	12-Rep Max Weight plus 10-15 lb.		6-8	60
	Same		6-8	60
	Same		6-8	60
_____	Same		6-8	0
Tricep Exercise	12-Rep Max Weight plus 10-15 lb.		6-8	60
	Same		6-8	60
	Same		6-8	60
_____	Same		6-8	0
Bicep Exercise	12-Rep Max Weight plus 10-15 lb.		6-8	60
	Same		6-8	60
	Same		6-8	60
_____	Same		6-8	0
Adbominal Exercise	12-Rep Max Weight plus 10-15 lb.		6-8	60
	Same		6-8	60
	Same		6-8	60
_____	Same		6-8	0

Stretches (Put a check when complete):	
Chest	√
Back	√
Shoulder	√
Tricep	√
Bicep	√
Abdominal	√
Total Workout Time:	45 minutes

Completed Program			
Date:			
Warm up:			
	Weight	Reps	Seconds Between Sets
Chest Exercise _____			
Back Exercise _____			
Shoulder Exercise _____			
Tricep Exercise _____			
Bicep Exerclse _____			
Adbominal Exercise _____			

Stretches (Put a check when complete):

Chest	
Back	
Shoulder	
Tricep	
Bicep	
Abdominal	
Total Workout Time:	

After working out, how do I feel emotionally? Physically?

FIRST STEPS TO FITNESS RESISTANCE PROGRAM
Week Three Lower Body

Before I start, how do I feel physically? Emotionally?

Planned Program				
Date:		Warm up:		
	Formula for Amount of Weight	Weight	Reps	Seconds Between Sets
Glute Exercise	12-Rep Max Weight plus 10-15 lb.		6-8	60
	Same		6-8	60
	Same		6-8	60
_____	Same		6-8	0
Quadricep Exercise	12-Rep Max Weight plus 10-15 lb.		6-8	60
	Same		6-8	60
	Same		6-8	60
_____	Same		6-8	0
Hamstring Exercise	12-Rep Max Weight plus 10-15 lb.		6-8	60
	Same		6-8	60
	Same		6-8	60
_____	Same		6-8	0
Inner Thigh Exercise	12-Rep Max Weight plus 10-15 lb.		6-8	60
	Same		6-8	60
	Same		6-8	60
_____	Same		6-8	0
Outer Thigh Exercise	12-Rep Max Weight plus 10-15 lb.		6-8	60
	Same		6-8	60
	Same		6-8	60
_____	Same		6-8	0
Calf Exercise	12-Rep Max Weight plus 10-15 lb.		6-8	60
	Same		6-8	60
	Same		6-8	60
_____	Same		6-8	0
Abdominal Exercise	12-Rep Max Weight plus 10-15 lb.		6-8	60
	Same		6-8	60
	Same		6-8	60
_____	Same		6-8	0
Lower Back Exercise	12-Rep Max Weight plus 10-15 lb.		6-8	60
	Same		6-8	60
	Same		6-8	60
_____	Same		6-8	0

Stretches (Put a check when complete):	
Glute	√
Quadricep	√
Hamstring	√
Inner & Outer Thigh	√
Calf	√
Abdominal & Lower Back	√
Total Workout Time:	45 minutes

Completed Program		
Date:		Warm up:
	Weight	Reps	Seconds Between Sets

Glute Exercise			
_____			

Quadricep Exercise			
_____			

Hamstring Exercise			
_____			

Inner Thigh Exercise			
_____			

Outer Thigh Exercise			
_____			

Calf Exercise			
_____			

Abdominal Exercise			
_____			

Lower Back Exercise			
_____			

Stretches (Put a check when complete):

Glute	
Quadricep	
Hamstring	
Inner & Outer Thigh	
Calf	
Abdominal & Lower Back	
Total Workout Time:	

After working out, how do I feel emotionally? Physically?

FIRST STEPS TO FITNESS RESISTANCE PROGRAM
Week Four Upper Body

Before I start, how do I feel physically? Emotionally?

Planned Program					
Date:			Warm up:		
	Formula for Amount of Weight	Weight	Reps	Seconds Between Sets	
Chest Exercise	12-Rep Max Weight plus 15-20 lb.		4-6	60	
	Same		4-6	60	
	Same		4-6	60	
	Same		4-6	60	
_____	Same		4-6	0	
Back Exercise	12-Rep Max Weight plus 15-20 lb.		4-6	60	
	Same		4-6	60	
	Same		4-6	60	
	Same		4-6	60	
_____	Same		4-6	0	
Shoulder Exercise	12-Rep Max Weight plus 15-20 lb.		4-6	60	
	Same		4-6	60	
	Same		4-6	60	
	Same		4-6	60	
_____	Same		4-6	0	
Tricep Exercise	12-Rep Max Weight plus 15-20 lb.		4-6	60	
	Same		4-6	60	
	Same		4-6	60	
	Same		4-6	60	
_____	Same		4-6	0	
Bicep Exercise	12-Rep Max Weight plus 15-20 lb.		4-6	60	
	Same		4-6	60	
	Same		4-6	60	
	Same		4-6	60	
_____	Same		4-6	0	
Abdominal Exercise	12-Rep Max Weight plus 15-20 lb.		4-6	60	
	Same		4-6	60	
	Same		4-6	60	
	Same		4-6	60	
_____	Same		4-6	0	

Stretches (Put a check when complete):

Chest & Back	√
Shoulder	√
Tricep & Bicep	√
Abdominal	√
Total Workout Time:	54 minutes

Completed Program			
Date:			
Warm up:			
	Weight	Reps	Seconds Between Sets
Chest Exercise _____			
Back Exercise _____			
Shoulder Exercise _____			
Tricep Exercise _____			
Bicep Exercise _____			
Abdominal Exercise _____			

Stretches (Put a check when complete):

Chest & Back	
Shoulder	
Tricep & Bicep	
Abdominal	
Total Workout Time:	

After working out, how do I feel emotionally? Physically?

FIRST STEPS TO FITNESS RESISTANCE PROGRAM
Week Four Lower Body

Before I start, how do I feel physically? Emotionally?

Planned Program

	Formula for Amount of Weight	Weight	Reps	Seconds Between Sets
Date:		Warm up:		
Glute Exercise	12-Rep Max Weight plus 15-20 lb.		4-6	60
	Same		4-6	60
	Same		4-6	60
	Same		4-6	60
_____	Same		4-6	0
Quadricep Exercise	12-Rep Max Weight plus 15-20 lb.		4-6	60
	Same		4-6	60
	Same		4-6	60
	Same		4-6	60
_____	Same		4-6	0
Hamstring Exercise	12-Rep Max Weight plus 15-20 lb.		4-6	60
	Same		4-6	60
	Same		4-6	60
	Same		4-6	60
_____	Same		4-6	0
Inner Thigh Exercise	12-Rep Max Weight plus 15-20 lb.		4-6	60
	Same		4-6	60
	Same		4-6	60
	Same		4-6	60
_____	Same		4-6	0
Outer Thigh Exercise	12-Rep Max Weight plus 15-20 lb.		4-6	60
	Same		4-6	60
	Same		4-6	60
	Same		4-6	60
_____	Same		4-6	0
Calf Exercise	12-Rep Max Weight plus 15-20 lb.		4-6	60
	Same		4-6	60
	Same		4-6	60
	Same		4-6	60
_____	Same		4-6	0
Abdominal Exercise	12-Rep Max Weight plus 15-20 lb.		4-6	60
	Same		4-6	60
	Same		4-6	60
	Same		4-6	60
_____	Same		4-6	0
Lower Back Exercise	12-Rep Max Weight plus 15-20 lb.		4-6	60
	Same		4-6	60
	Same		4-6	60
	Same		4-6	60
_____	Same		4-6	0

Stretches (Put a check when complete):	
Glute & Calf	√
Quad & Ham	√
Inner & Outer Thigh	√
Abdominal & Lower Back	√
Total Workout Time:	54 minutes

Completed Program			
Date:			
Warm up:			
	Weight	Reps	Seconds Between Sets
Glute Exercise _____			
Quadricep Exercise _____			
Hamstring Exercise _____			
Inner Thigh Exercise _____			
Outer Thigh Exercise _____			
Calf Exercise _____			
Abdominal Exercise _____			
Lower Back Exercise _____			

Stretches (Put a check when complete):	
Glute & Calf	
Quad & Ham	
Inner & Outer Thigh	
Abdominal & Lower Back	
Total Workout Time:	

After working out, how do I feel emotionally? Physically?

MEASUREMENT CHART

Date/Time:	1.	2.		3.		4.		5.		6.	
Measurement			+ –		+ –		+ –		+ –		+ –
Chest											
Left Arm											
Right Arm											
Abs (Belly Button)											
Hip/Buttocks											
Left Leg											
Right Leg											
Left Calf											
Right Calf											
Total (+/-)											

MEASUREMENT CHART

Date/Time:	7.		8.		9		10.		11.		12.	
Measurement		+ −		+ −		+ −		+ −		+ −		+ −
Chest												
Left Arm												
Right Arm												
Abs (Belly Button)												
Hip/Buttocks												
Left Leg												
Right Leg												
Left Calf												
Right Calf												
Total (+/-)												

DAILY EATING PLAN

Planned Program

Date:	

MEAL ONE

Time	Food & Amounts	Calories	Fiber	Water
Breakfast				
	Total:			

MEAL TWO

Time	Food & Amounts	Calories	Fiber	Water
Snack				
	Total:			

MEAL THREE

Time	Food & Amounts	Calories	Fiber	Water
Lunch				
	Total:			

MEAL FOUR

Time	Food & Amounts	Calories	Fiber	Water
Snack				
	Total:			

MEAL FIVE

Time	Food & Amounts	Calories	Fiber	Water
Dinner				
	Total:			

PLANNED

Total Daily Meals	Total Daily Calories	Total Daily Fiber	Total Daily Water

Completed Program				
Date:				
MEAL ONE				
Time	Food & Amounts	Calories	Fiber	Water
Breakfast				
	Total:			
MEAL TWO				
Time	Food & Amounts	Calories	Fiber	Water
Snack				
	Total:			
MEAL THREE				
Time	Food & Amounts	Calories	Fiber	Water
Lunch				
	Total:			
MEAL FOUR				
Time	Food & Amounts	Calories	Fiber	Water
Snack				
	Total:			
MEAL FIVE				
Time	Food & Amounts	Calories	Fiber	Water
Dinner				
	Total:			
COMPLETED				

Total Daily Meals	Total Daily Calories	Total Daily Fiber	Total Daily Water

ACTION GOALS

Cardiovascular Goals:	Weekly	Monthly	Quarterly	Yearly
Type of aerobic workout				
How many days and how long you will work out				
Other aerobic goals				
Strength Goals:				
Type of strength workout				
How many days and how long you will work out				
Other strength goals				
Flexibility Goals:				
Type of flexibility workout				
How many days and how long you will work out				
Other flexibility goals				
Diet/Water Goals:				
Type of diet and water goals				
How many days you will follow your diet/water plan				
Other diet/water goals				
Miscellaneous Goals:				
Other action goals:				

RESULTS GOALS				
	Weekly	Monthly	Quarterly	Yearly
Weight				
Inches/ Measurements				
Body Fat				
Other				

SCHEDULE SHEET

WEEK		MON.	TUES.	WED.	THURS.	FRI.	SAT.	SUN.	Weekly Goals	Weekly Rewards
WEEK 1	WORK-OUT TYPE									
	MEAL PLAN									
WEEK 2	WORK-OUT TYPE									
	MEAL PLAN									

SCHEDULE SHEET

WEEK		MON.	TUES.	WED.	THURS.	FRI.	SAT.	SUN.	Weekly Goals	Weekly Rewards
WEEK 3	WORK-OUT TYPE									
	MEAL PLAN									
WEEK 4	WORK-OUT TYPE									
	MEAL PLAN									

Monthly Goals:		Quarterly Goals:		Annual Goals:	
Monthly Rewards:		Quarterly Rewards:		Annual Rewards:	

Positive Replacement Template

I _____ today.

I am in the process of _____ today.

Because I am patient, hardworking, and committed, I am

_____.

Positive Replacement Template

I _____ today.

I am in the process of _____ today.

Because I am patient, hardworking, and committed, I am

_____.

Positive Replacement Template

I _____ today.

I am in the process of _____ today.

Because I am patient, hardworking, and committed, I am

_____.

Index

About the Author

In addition to earning a bachelor's degree in human services with emphases in psychology and sociology from the University of Nebraska at Omaha, Elizabeth Williams has earned several fitness instructor certifications, including International Sports Science Association (ISSA) Personal Trainer, ISSA Fitness Therapist, and Aerobics and Fitness Association of America (AFAA) Primary Group Exercise Certification. She has also successfully completed continuing education courses in nutrition, stress management, senior fitness, and flexibility, among others.

As a personal trainer specializing in the overweight female population, Elizabeth has trained hundreds of clients. As an area manager for a fitness company, she interviewed and worked with hundreds of personal trainers. It was through this work with clients and trainers as well as her own personal struggles with fitness and body image that the concepts for *The First Steps to Fitness* were born and tested.

Elizabeth lives in Sacramento, California, with her husband, Mike, and son, Jake. She is currently working on her next book.

Fitness Notebook